Expectant Blessings

Expectant Blessings

Prayers, Poems, and Devotions for You and Your Baby

SUSANNA FOTH AUGHTMON

WORTHY*
Inspired

Published by Worthy Inspired, an imprint of Worthy Publishing Group, a division of Worthy Media, Inc., One Franklin Park, 6100 Tower Circle, Suite 210, Franklin, TN 37067.

WORTHY is a registered trademark of Worthy Media, Inc.

HELPING PEOPLE EXPERIENCE THE HEART OF GOD

eBook available wherever digital books are sold.

Names: Aughtmon, Susanna Foth, 1970- author.
Title: Praise for expectant blessings : prayers, poems, and devotions for you and your baby / Susanna Foth Aughtmon.
Description: Franklin, TN : Praise Worthy Publishing, 2016. | Includes bibliographical references and index.
Identifiers: LCCN 2015045849 | ISBN 9781617956683 (tradepaper : alk. paper)
Subjects: LCSH: Pregnant women--Prayers and devotions. | Pregnant women--Religious life.
Classification: LCC BV4846 .A79 2016 | DDC 242/.6431--dc23
LC record available at http://lccn.loc.gov/2015045849

Scripture quotations are from THE HOLY BIBLE, NEW INTERNATIONAL VERSION®, NIV® Copyright © 1973, 1978, 1984 by Biblica, Inc.® Used by permission. All rights reserved worldwide.

ISBN 978-1-61795-668-3

Cover Design: Jeff Jansen/Aesthetic Soup
Cover Photo: Ashley Jade
Photograph used with permission from Emy+Annie |emyandannie.com
Additional Cover Photos: iStockphoto.com

Printed in the United States of America
1 2 3 4 5 6—WOR—20 19 18 17 16

This book is dedicated to
Jack, Will, and Addison . . .
the three beautiful, large-headed baby boys
who made me a mom.
Being your mom has turned my heart
inside out with joy.
I am so proud of the young men
that you are becoming.
Know that Dad and I love you the most.

Contents

Introduction

PREGNANCY IS one of the most beautiful adventures to be had in a woman's life. The experience of growing a new little person is an amazing, awe-inspiring season of life. God is at work in you both physically and spiritually as He crafts this baby in your belly. The amount of love and hope that flood your heart for this little one during this process will leave you changed forever. From the sighting of the blue lines on that pregnancy test, the transformation has begun. You are a mom. Now and forevermore.

I have had the great privilege of growing three new little people: Jack, Will, and Addison. Lovebugs, every one. Each time I discovered I was pregnant, I was so overwhelmed I cried. So much joy! So much hope! (And then there was also the nausea and wild hormone fluctuations . . . but those brought different kinds of tears.) My husband, Scott, and I were beyond thrilled at the prospect of being parents. I couldn't get over the fact that I was this lucky, this blessed, to be able to bring a new little one into the world. And I absolutely could not wait to be a mom to these little ones. I was especially hoping they were chubby . . . because I do so love chubby babies. I got my wish all three times. So. Chubby.

Each of my pregnancies was completely different. Each of them took place in a time of transition for our family. My first pregnancy took place when we were youth pastors at a new church. My second took place during our move to the East Coast. And my third pregnancy took place during our first year church planting back on the West Coast. For some reason babies and transition seemed to go hand in hand for us. And God used those transitions coupled with the promise of new life to bring us closer to Him. The vulnerability of being in a new situation showed us time and again how much we needed Him—His grace, His love, His provision, and His guidance. What we wanted more than anything . . . along with a healthy newborn with squeezable thighs . . . was for this little one to be close to God, too.

God always wants to pull us closer to His heart. And pregnancy is a wonderfully unique time for that to occur. A new life is being created. The Creator of the Universe is inviting you to get in on the joy of it. He wants to grow your little one, but He also wants to grow your heart. He doesn't just want to shape your child's ten fingers and ten toes; He wants to shape your soul. There is no bigger transformation that you will experience than becoming a mom. Whether it is your first amazing pregnancy or your seventh amazing pregnancy, there is always more joy, more love, more hope, more wonder to be had as this new life grows within you.

When I found out I was going to be a mom for the first time, I truly could not contain myself. Becoming a new mom consumed me. I talked about it. I dreamt about it. I wrote about it. All of the poems in this little book were written from my mother's heart and born out of my mommy's desire to connect with my unborn baby during my first pregnancy. I was so amazed by the miracle that was taking place inside of my body, I tried to capture my feelings and emotions in words and phrases, syllables and rhyme. I knew that no amount of prose could capture the love and overwhelming sense of awe that filled me as I watched my body change and grow. But it seemed right to keep trying. The more I talked to my babies and the more I sang to them, the closer I felt to them. The more I prayed and asked God's richest blessings over them, the closer I felt to God.

This moment, when new life is welling up within you, is the perfect time to get closer to the One who loves you the most. To reach out to Him. To connect with Him. To trust Him through the ins and outs of this amazing season. Each of the devotions in this book were written in hopes that you would laugh, be encouraged, and know that the God of the Universe holds you in the palm of His hand during your entire pregnancy. Each Scripture included is a reminder of His truth and His deep love for you. Each prayer is simply a jumping-off place for you to start a conversation with the One who loves you and your little one the most. And the biggest hope of all is that the thoughts and prayers and poems found in this book will be a blessing to you and to your baby.

So in the spirit of Jesus, who felt it was truly important to bless the little ones in His life, may you have a truly wonderful pregnancy as you bless this sweet baby.

Chapter 1

This Is It!

THIS IS IT! Your moment has arrived. You are pregnant. A mom-to-be. A soon-to-be-nesting mama bird, as it were. Unbelievable, isn't it? So let the praying commence. Because that is what we moms do. We hope. We dream. We peruse baby websites, and we pray.

You may not think that you know how to pray, but prayers are just conversations that you have with your heavenly Father. It makes sense that you would put your questions, your deep concerns, your greatest hopes, and your innermost thoughts to the One who loves you and this little one most of all. He has the power and ability to do amazing things.

God wants to be close to you whether or not you are pregnant. But there is something so revelatory about having a baby that it seems to invite His presence even more. You are experiencing daily miracles, and He wants in on that. All the joy. All the hope. All the creativity. And you need Him right now. In those moments of reading His Word and listening for His voice, He will remind you once again how much He delights in this new little one that He is forming.

My prayers during pregnancy took on a third-party aspect. Whatever prayers that I prayed were witnessed by me, my heavenly Father, and my baby. Jesus said, "When two or three gather in my name, I am with them." For the next nine months, I had a constant prayer partner on hand to agree with me. When my husband, Scott, joined in we had a real prayer meeting going on.

Now, you may not be a very long-winded pray-er. That is okay. Prayers can be real and to the point. Like, "Dear Jesus, where are the Tums? I need them now." It is an important prayer. Anti-nausea prayers are mostly short laments like "Help." And "Sweet Mercy." And then there are those moments when the greatness of all that is taking place inside of you will lift your heart so high, that all you can do is say, "Thank You. Thank You. Thank You." The beauty of prayer is that it is spirit talking to Spirit. Deep talking to deep. God knows all that is contained in your heart when you pray.

My good friend, Pastor Mark, says that even after we leave this earth, the prayers we pray go on and on into eternity. So while you may forget the prayers that you have prayed over this sweet one, the One who placed the stars in the universe, gathers them close and continues answering those prayers as the years pass by. So now is the time to pray big. Get creative. Pray for this baby in every possible way that you can think of. For anything and everything that God lays upon your heart to pray. And know, beyond a shadow of a doubt, that He is already answering.

Lord,
I am overwhelmed by Your goodness.
Thank You for answering my prayers.
Show me how to love and pray for this little one.
Thank You for the gift of this new life.
Amen.

He said to them,
"Let the little children come to me, and do not hinder them,
for the kingdom of God belongs to such as these.
Truly I tell you, anyone who will not receive
the kingdom of God like a little child
will never enter it."
And he took the children in his arms,
put his hands on them and blessed them.

—

Mark 10:14–16

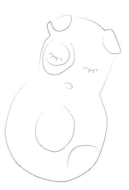

Chapter 2

The Pregnant Path

FINDING OUT that you are pregnant is one of the most life-altering, beautiful things that can ever happen to you. In that moment, you became a part of a miracle. The divine and the ordinary collide. A new person is coming to life, being knit together, by the love and providence of God, inside of you. This is all at once fantastic and terrifying. You may burst into tears or jump up and down, laughing with the joy of it. Or you may do both at the same time. This is perfectly normal behavior during pregnancy.

The first time I found out I was pregnant, I screamed so loudly I completely freaked out my husband. This is not the best way to announce your pregnancy. It would have been a good idea to tell him beforehand, "Honey, I am taking a pregnancy test right now." At least this is what he told me after he recovered from his near heart attack. It wasn't that I didn't want to include him in the special moment. It's just that I wasn't expecting the test to turn up positive. I had taken a lot of pregnancy tests over our five years of marriage. I wasn't sure that I could actually get pregnant. And then here I was seeing that I

WAS pregnant and I was undone. I didn't have any words to describe my feelings. Just piercing screams of joy.

It is a rare day when you realize that the course of your life has just shifted. The day you find out you are heading down the pregnant path is a day to remember and ponder in your heart. (It is surely one that my husband will never forget.) And after you have pondered this wondrous event, go ahead and do some deep breathing exercises. You are about to launch into an adventure in the unknown.

The pregnant path is a journey of waiting. Hoping. And trusting. The trust part is huge. Looking down at your positive pregnancy test, you have a choice. You can choose to (a) freak out or (b) trust the One who loves you most of all to walk this journey with you. He will understand if you freak out . . . but He would really love for you to trust Him—wholly and completely. You should know that the beauty of trusting in your heavenly Father is understanding that even though you are not in control of this experience . . . He is.

He had this little one in mind for you before you ever did. Despite what you may think, He was not surprised when your test registered two blue lines. Trust Him and know that He is walking down your pregnant path with you. He is more in love with your little baby than you are. If you let Him, He will show you all the pleasure that is to be had during this season of your life.

Lord,
I trust in You. In Your wisdom.
In Your goodness. In Your faithfulness.
I know that this baby is a part of
Your plan for my life.
Thank You for leading me in Your ways.
Amen.

I'm Expecting You!

Describe how you found out you were pregnant
and how you felt.

_____

_____

_____

_____

_____

_____

_____

_____

_____

_____

_____

_____

_____

_____

_____

_____

_____

Baby's Due Date: _____

Chapter 3

All This Joy

JOY IS A HUGE PART of being a new mom. If this pregnancy has been a long-awaited event, you might want to prepare the people around you for the onset of all the happy that you will be exuding. If you have been longing for a little one, it completely makes sense that you would break into cheery songs of praise and pregnant jigs at the news. Just keep the jigs on the less-rambunctious side. You should know that there are going to be moments when you will burst into tears because of all the hope welling up within you. You will experience your heart cracking open with love in a way that it never has before. New life is taking place inside of you. The joy just keeps coming. Does it get any better than this? I don't think so.

Now . . . there is also the possibility that your pregnancy was completely unplanned and you are thinking, *What in the world? Happy isn't exactly where I am living right now.* But there is still room for joy, even amidst the chaotic emotions. Mary, Jesus' mom, had the craziest surprise pregnancy ever. She couldn't believe that she was going to be a mom, let alone a mom to God's Son. She was completely freaked out and had every right to be. And yet in those moments of confusion and fear, she started to sing. A song of praise. Because she realized that God had ordained this. This was her new journey. He was blessing her. She didn't understand it, but she was going with it.

This is your new journey, too. God is pouring out His blessing on you in the form of this little one. Whether you realize it or not, this baby is an answer to your prayers. The One who knows you, the Giver of every perfect gift, knows exactly what you need. And in this moment in time? This baby is part of that. Even if it feels overwhelming. Even if the timing seems crazy. (In case you were wondering . . . there is no perfect time to have a baby.) Even if you are a little scared and are overwhelmed by nausea . . . go with the joy. Share the joy with the ones you love. Throw back your head and sing. With one hand on your belly and one hand on your heart, tell the One who loves you so much how much you love Him back.

Lord,
Thank You for Your overwhelming joy!
Thank You for this new life that You are
blessing me with. You are an amazing God,
full of good surprises. I love You.
Amen.

For You, Baby

I'm dreaming dreams of you, baby,
Each night when I lie in bed, I dream a thousand
dreams of you
      Dreams of a brown boy or a rosy girl
      With Daddy's eyes and Mommy's nose
      Butter soft skin and round chubby legs
      Safe in my arms and close to my heart
I can't help thinking that my sweetest dreams are of you, baby.

I'm thinking thoughts of you, baby,
Each morning when I wake up, I think a thousand thoughts
of you
      Thoughts of your moods and of your smiles
      The sound of your giggles and sad little cries
      The smell of your skin after a warm morning bath
      Safe in my arms and filling my mind
I can't help thinking that my purest thoughts are of you, baby.

I'm hoping hopes for you, baby,
Each afternoon as I sit in the sun, I hope a thousand hopes
for you
      Hopes for blue mornings and rainy afternoons
      For dreams come true and wishes granted

For love and goodness and peace and mercy to
surround you
Safe in my arms and hugged to my chest
I can't help thinking that my highest hopes are for you, baby.

I'm wondering wonders about you, baby,
Each twilight as I look out my window, I wonder a thousand
wonders about you
    Wonders of will you be a hand holder or a cheek kisser?
    Will you like ice cream? Will you catch bugs?
    And how many times can I squeeze you in one day?
    Safe in my arms and near to my soul
I can't help thinking that my loftiest wonders are of you, baby.

I'm praying prayers for you, baby,
Each evening as I stare into the heavens, I pray a thousand
prayers for you
    Prayers of joy and protection
    Of grace and endless forgiveness
    Of wisdom and patience and blessing and faith
    Safe in His arms and bundled in His Spirit
I can't help thinking that my loudest prayers are for you, baby.

And I can't help knowing, baby, that you are the answer to my
prayers.

Chapter 4

Spreading the Good News

THERE ARE ONLY a few times in your life when the information you hold, can make the people who love you absolutely lose their minds. One of those times is when you tell them that you are having a baby. There may be some screaming. Some disbelief. Some tears of joy. If you are telling the person face-to-face, you can expect some ecstatic hugging. Possibly some jumping up and down. This is seriously fantastic news that you are sharing. The world as they know it is about to get better. Someone whom they love is having another someone whom they love. It just does not get any better than that.

One of the best calls that I ever made was when Scott and I called to tell his grandmother Alice, aka Granny, that we were expecting our first baby. Granny was in New York visiting relatives for the summer. She was a little hard of hearing so I was pretty much yelling into the phone. "Granny?" "Sue?" "Yes! It's me, Sue. Scott and I are calling because we have something fun to tell you." "What is it?" "We are going to have a baby." "What?" "We are going to have a baby!" "You're up the flue?" "What?" "Up the flue! You're pregnant?" "Yes! We are pregnant

. . . what did you call it again?" "Up the flue!" "Okay . . . I am up the flue!" I am pretty sure that "up the flue" is a saying from the 1920s . . . but we were going with it. Granny got so happy, she started laughing and crying and wheezing a little. She always wheezed when she laughed. It was one of the best sounds I had ever heard in my life.

Sharing the joy of becoming a parent with those you love is important because pregnancy is a shared journey. The reason that your people are so excited to hear about your pregnancy is because they are already invested . . . in you. They love YOU. And this baby is an extension of you. Your parents, grandparents, and friends embark on a journey of loving this little one as soon as they find out he is coming. You have heard the saying "It takes a village to raise a child." Well, these folks are your village. You have their collective wisdom, help, and love to draw on once this baby is born. You have their support and their encouragement to lean on throughout these next nine months.

Family and friends are a gift that your heavenly Father has given you. You may not have two nickels to rub together, but if you have people who love you and your baby, you are rich. Loving each other was His idea. When you love and are loved by those around you, you are fulfilling your heavenly Father's heart's desire. He is over the moon about this baby. He wants everyone else to be, too. So soak up the joy telling your people and making those calls and know that your heavenly Father is right in the middle of it. He loves good news.

Lord,
Thank You for the joy of this good news I get to share.
Thank You for the people who love me
and love this baby.
And thank You, most of all, for being right
in the middle of this joy.
Amen.

Good News!

Describe how you announced to your family and friends that you were pregnant.

Chapter 5

Great Expectations

EXPECTATIONS ARE A HUGE PART of pregnancy. You are *expecting* a new wonderful addition to your family. You are *expecting* an adorable little one who will light up your life with joy. And you are *expecting* for this season of life to go well. What you may not be *expecting* are some of the surprises that pregnancy can spring on you along the way.

During my pregnancies, I experienced a great deal of nausea. My mom never had morning sickness. So I expected that I would be blessed with her wonderful nausea-free DNA. It was not to be. I became best friends with sea bands and saltine crackers. Strong smells sent me right over the edge. I could smell garlic from a mile away. The pregnancy I *expected* was not the pregnancy I got. And I am not the only one who has felt that way.

One of my good friends experienced some surprises during her second pregnancy. When she showed me a picture of her sonogram, I remember saying, "This is so exciting . . . wait . . . WHAT? Are you having twins?" With a kind of dazed smile she said, "Yes! It's twins! Can you believe it?" And I could not believe it. And she could not believe it. Two babies. Double the crazy. Double the joy. That takes the unexpected to a whole new level.

In the next nine months, you may have a smidge of the unexpected come your way. The reality of what your pregnancy is like may not match up to your idea of what you thought it would be. But that is okay. The growing of a new life has a way of changing everything . . . from your eating habits to your emotional state. When you find yourself disappointed because something is not going exactly the way that you thought it would? Try and do those deep breathing exercises . . . and then go with it. Let go of your expectations, whatever they are, and send up this prayer, "Lord, I wasn't expecting this . . . AT ALL . . . but I know that this isn't a surprise for You. And I am choosing to trust You in this." This is the kind of prayer that will let you breathe.

Expectations, in and of themselves, are hit or miss. But even though you may be walking out a different pregnancy than you expected, one expectation will be met without a doubt. God will be with you. Whatever surprises your pregnancy brings you, whether it is nausea or twins or both, He is near. Whether you are having an unexpected moment of joy or an unexpected moment of craziness, He will hem you in on every side. And He will surround you and your little one with His all-encompassing love in the coming days. Those are some great expectations to have realized.

Lord,
Each morning when I wake up,
You remind me of Your new mercies.
You hem me in with Your love and grace.
Thank You for exceeding all my expectations.
Amen.

You Are God's Child

You are His little lamb
You are His precious coin
You are His tender branch
You are God's child

He is your Shepherd strong
He is your Caretaker
He is your One True Vine
You are God's child

You are His ray of sun
You are His love on earth
You are His pride and joy
You are God's child

He is your Prince of Peace
He is your Only Way
He is your Life and Truth
You are God's child

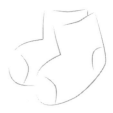

Chapter 6

His Little One

YOU MAY BE completely surprised by how protective you are now that you are a mom-to-be. You might become hyper-vigilant about avoiding food that could be unhealthy for your little one. You may start taking your vitamins religiously and exercising like you never have before. You may even change your driving habits and try to stay within the speed limit now. It is an amazing transformation that takes place. I was truly unprepared for how territorial I would become as an expect-ant mom. This baby . . . was mine. And Scott's, of course . . . but mine. And that being said, I was a mommy on a mission. Taking care of baby. Go-cart riding and gymnastics were a thing of the past. (Okay . . . so the last time I rode a go-cart I was twelve, and my gymnastics skills were limited to a very shaky-looking cartwheel . . . but I was done with them forever.) I wanted to do everything possible to keep this little one safe.

Every mom should take the best possible care of herself and her baby. But you should know that you have a way more powerful line of defense in protecting this little one than you can possibly imagine. This isn't just your baby to guard and protect. Someone else has a vested interest in this little one. That is his Creator. Your baby is really His baby. You have been given the enormous privilege of being this little one's parent. But his heavenly Father is the One who is really calling the shots. He is the One who is truly vigilant about guarding this sweet baby night and day from all harm.

You can take a deep breath and know, in the deepest part of your heart, that this baby's Creator, the One who loves him most of all, is his true guardian. He is protecting him and keeping him safe in ways that you couldn't even begin to hope or imagine. He is keeping watch over him because He loves him so very much. He will do so from now until the end of his days. He promises you this in His Word because this baby is His baby. Let His peace flood your heart, knowing that He is protecting your little one. And always will.

Lord,
Thank You for the miracle of this baby.
I am so glad that You care for him
even more than I do.
I commit this precious baby to Your care.
Amen.

For you created my inmost being;
you knit me together in my mother's womb.
I praise you because I am fearfully and wonderfully made;
your works are wonderful,
I know that full well.
My frame was not hidden from you
when I was made in the secret place.
When I was woven together in the depths of the earth,
your eyes saw my unformed body.
All the days ordained for me were written in your book
before one of them came to be.

—

Psalm 139:13–16

Chapter 7

Finding Your People

PREGNANCY IS an all-hands-on-deck time of life. You are probably used to taking care of yourself. You may not want to bother people with your needs or put them out. This is understandable, but this may not be the best time to be thinking this way. You have a choice. You can try and get through these next nine months on your own. Or you can find your people.

My cousin Gretchen and her one-year-old, Jakob, came with me to the doctor's office for my first visit. After trying to get pregnant for so long, I couldn't quite believe it was really happening. A nurse had me take a pregnancy test. Then I sat in an exam room with hands folded, waiting for the official verdict. She poked her head back in and said, "Yes, Mrs. Aughtmon, you are pregnant. We will see you back here in a few weeks for your first prenatal checkup. You can go out and set up your next appointment with the receptionist."

I nodded and then I began to cry. The nurse, taking it all in, stepped inside and put her arm around my shoulders. She gave me a squeeze and said, "Oh, honey . . . it's so good, isn't it?" And it was so good. The realized hope. And the kind words and hug from a stranger. As I walked into the waiting room, Gretchen joined me in my happy tears and said, "Jakob, Auntie Suz is pregnant! You are going to have a cousin!" I had found two of my people. Cousin Gretchen and the nurse. They celebrated with me and recognized the importance of the moment I was experiencing.

Your people are the people who will support you, rejoice with you, and lift you up during these next nine months. Some of these people you already know. Some you may find along the way. They are the ones who cry tears of joy with you when you tell them you are pregnant. They are the people who say that they can't wait to squeeze the precious baby and see if she possibly has your eyebrows. These are the folks whom you can lean on. They will be happy to bring you a meal on a particularly nauseous day, go to a checkup with you, or if you already have a few little ones running around, watch them for you so that you can grab a nap.

God has placed people in your life to encourage you on the long pregnant path, to help you when you feel overwhelmed, and to celebrate with you in moments of joy. Recognizing that you need others is not a sign of weakness . . . it is a sign of wisdom. You were created with community in mind. For being with others. For building each other up and leaning on each other. For loving each other. Finding your people is just one more of the heavenly Father's gifts you will get to experience during this beautiful journey.

Lord,
You are too wonderful for words.
I am so grateful for Your care and
encouragement during this journey.
Thank You that You show Your love for me
through the people who surround me.
Amen.

The First Hello

Early this morning
Birds were chirping outside windows
A fluttery breeze blew the leaves up and down streets
And the sun broke through the misty clouds to warm the earth.

Early this morning
Showers and baths steamed up mirrors
Teeth were brushed and hair was combed.
And a million outfits were picked out for a new day.

Early this morning
Coffeepots were brewing and teapots were whistling
Toasts were toasting and jam was jamming
And a million breakfasts were prepared to fill hungry tummies.

Early this morning
People got in cars, buses, and trains to go to work
Storekeepers opened their doors for business
And a million children bundled themselves up to go to school.

Early this morning
Graces and praises went up to heavens
Petitions and prayers made their way into eternity
And a million thankful songs were lifted up to God the Creator.

Early this morning
As I lay on my belly in my bed
I felt a small tap, the tiniest nudge, the sweetest flutter
And a million tears sprang to my eyes as you said your
first hello.

Hello baby.

Chapter 8

A Pregnant Meditation

PREGNANCY IS a time of life that invites a lot of deep thinking. So much is going on in your body and in your heart, you can't help but get caught up thinking, *What in the world is going on inside of me?* and *Why can't I stop crying?* and *I never knew I could be so hot . . . can someone turn on the air conditioner?* These thoughts are followed by more thoughts about your little one. *Is she growing enough?*, *When will I start feeling her move?*, and *What does she look like?* You are constantly thinking and pondering the myriad of different issues that surround pregnancy.

Meditation is one way that you can gather your thoughts and bring about a little peace of mind amidst all of your worries and questions. You may picture meditation as a practice of sitting cross-legged on the floor, emptying your mind and trying to get as relaxed as possible. But the kind of meditation that the Bible encourages is the practice of mulling over a portion of God's Word and chewing on it, while getting every little morsel of truth and nuance of hope out of it. It is a steady filling of the mind with the wonder and powerful truth of who God is and how much He loves you.

A wonderful psalm to meditate on is Psalm 139. The fact that God knit you together in your mother's womb. That you are fearfully and wonderfully made. The fact that He is, right now, knitting your little baby together in your womb. Let the glory of it all seep into your mind and color your thoughts for the rest of your day. Keep reading on in the psalm. It just gets better and better.

Did you know that God is going before and following behind you? That He sees all your comings and goings? That there is nowhere that you can go that He cannot find you? It really is too much for us to take in, isn't it? All that love. All that goodness. All that care found in the arms of the One who creates galaxies with a word. It is the truth. Chew on this for a while: All the days ordained for you were written in His book before one of them came to be. Even this day. He knew it would come to pass. He wants you to know that. And there it is. That beautiful peace of His that passes all understanding when you rest in His truth and meditate on His Word. It doesn't get any better than that.

Lord,
Thank You for this growing baby who is inside me.
As he grows, help me to meditate more and
more on Your truth, filling my mind with
Your love and goodness.
Thank You for the joy of experiencing
growth in a new way.
Amen.

Friend of Jesus Prayer

Dear Jesus,
Thank You for this sweet baby.
Thank You that You have created him
to be a unique individual,
complete with his own personality and sense of humor.
Thank You that You have thoughts and plans
and desires for him
and that You want to be a part of his life.
I pray that this baby would be Your friend.
I pray that he would hear Your voice and know it.
I ask that he would be Your follower and Your disciple.
Even when he is small,
let him know that You love to be with him
and that You treasure him.
Bring people into his life who are lovers of You,
so that they can travel down Your path with him.
I commit this precious baby to Your care, Lord.
Thank You for the privilege of being this little one's mom.
Amen.

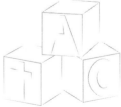

Chapter 9

Welcome to the Pregnant Moms Club!

YOU MAY NOT have realized it, but as soon as that little sweet pea began to grow inside of you, you joined a giant worldwide club that is growing every day. Club members hail from every tribe and every tongue. It is the Pregnant Moms Club. Pregnant moms everywhere give each other the all-knowing look that says, "I can tell that you are doing something life altering and amazing right now . . . me, too!" These people are your tribe. They will get you. Your weird cravings. Your mood swings. Your covetous feelings toward the latest stroller model. They are walking in your very pregnant shoes.

But one thing that you should understand is that the club members have a wide variety of pregnancy experiences. You may find that even though you have a lot of similarities with these women, you have just as many differences. And comparing your pregnancy with someone else's is not your best plan.

My sister-in-law, Cheri, was a glower. Pregnancy smiled upon her, and she just seemed to get cuter as the months went along. She was full of energy and goodwill in her early pregnancy. I was pregnant with my first when she was pregnant with her third. While I felt a little bit like I might die from all the nausea, I was a thrower-upper, I don't think Cheri ever threw up. Not once. It seemed unfair. But maybe if you asked Cheri she would say the same. She developed gestational diabetes the moment she got pregnant and had to give herself insulin shots in her tummy. Ouch. I never even had one shot. We each had our share of joys and difficulties. Pregnant life is like that.

It is easy to get drawn into comparisons in the Pregnant Moms Club. Whose pregnancy is easier? Who has cuter pants? Who gets maternity leave? Who is a glower and who is a thrower-upper? But the truth is, your pregnancy is completely your own. No two pregnancies are alike. Not even your own. Comparisons are useless, and to be honest, they are energy suckers.

God is doing a new work inside of you. He is molding in His image a human being who has never been molded before. He has you in the very set of circumstances that you were destined for. He is at work in you in a way that He never has been before. It is up to you to fully embrace it. The unfettered beauty of it and the hardship of it. The joy and the not-so-much-joy of it. When you do, you will find that your heavenly Father will flood you with grace for all the difficult moments and hope for the beauty that is to come. And that is something that all the club members are invited to experience.

Lord,
I am so thankful for this baby.
Thank You for the unique experience
of this pregnancy.
You are more than enough for me.
Amen.

Baby's Family

Mommy's Name: _____

Daddy's Name: _____

Siblings' Names and Ages: _____

_____

_____

Mommy's Work: _____

Daddy's Work: _____

Where We Live: _____

Our Family Story This Far: _____

_____

_____

_____

_____

_____

_____

_____

_____

_____

_____

_____

Chapter 10

Being Unafraid

YOU MAY BE one of those pregnant people who wants to know all the possibilities, both good and bad, that could take place during your pregnancy. Knowing this helps you feel prepared and more in control. Or you may be one of those pregnant people with an overactive imagination. And when you read up on all the conditions that could possibly happen during pregnancy, it pitches you headlong into an anxiety attack. Because you were already worried about the mechanics of breast feeding and fitting back into your pre-pregnancy pants, you weren't even thinking about the fact that something could happen to this tiny one growing inside of you. Thinking about that completely freaks you out.

When I found out that I was pregnant, I immediately went out and bought *a* best-selling pregnancy book to guide me through my three trimesters with wisdom and common sense. I don't know what I thought this book was going to say, but I got about three pages in before I started hyperventilating. It started describing assorted things that could go wrong early on in pregnancy. I began to imagine all sorts of different scenarios.

A few weeks later when I actually experienced spotting off and on, I was terrified. Fear can grow by leaps and bounds in mere moments. I was paralyzed by the thought of losing what I had just gained.

Being afraid isn't a bad thing; it is a human thing. Fear is also a normal part of being a mom. Because you love this baby SO much, you don't want anything to happen to him. You are in for nine months of not knowing exactly what is taking place in your uterus. That can be scary. You feel powerless. But you should know that the One who is forming this little one inside of you is all powerful.

Your heavenly Father is the One who is knitting this tiny baby together, molecule by molecule. He has a plan. He loves you. He loves this baby. And He can hold you both in a place of love no matter what is going on in your body or what the outcome of your pregnancy is. Your heavenly Father is inviting you to trust Him with this little one. No matter what. He is inviting you to believe in Him and know that surrounded by His love, grounded in His hope, and resting in His mercy, He holds both of you completely. In His presence, you can let your fears rest in the greatness of who He is and the all-encompassing love that He has for you. And He will never let you go.

Lord,
Thank You for knowing my fears,
for listening to my prayers, and for
intervening on my behalf.
Bring me closer and closer to You.
Thank You for being my Deliverer.
Amen.

The LORD watches over you—
the LORD is your shade at your right hand;
the sun will not harm you by day,
nor the moon by night.
The LORD will keep you from all harm—
he will watch over your life;
the LORD will watch over your coming and going
both now and forevermore.

—

Psalm 121:5–8

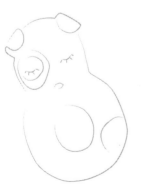

Chapter 11

Money Matters

THERE IS NOTHING like having a baby to make you take a serious look at your finances. You might experience the cruel shock of, "Wait. What? How much did you say raising a child was going to cost?" If you are really serious about financial planning, you can run the numbers from the cost of birthing someone all the way through funding college. And then after you regain consciousness, you might want to stick your fingers in your ears and say, "La-la-la-la-la-la . . . I can't hear what you are saying." This is denial. It works for some of us. It can be easy to be overwhelmed with the thought of providing well for your little one. But take another one of those deep breaths. You are not alone.

When I was pregnant with my first son, Jack, Scott and I were both working. My deepest desire was to be able to stay home with my baby. I was working at a start-up in Silicon Valley. But I started dreaming about the possibility of bringing in income while being Jack's main caregiver. Scott and I prayed about it. I started putting out feelers, telling my friends that I was going to start my own home decorating/organizing business. Within a month, I had several clients lined up. I wouldn't be making as much, but if Scott and I got creative with budgeting, we figured we could make it work.

We had a financial plan, but God had a better one. The day that I brought in my letter of resignation to my company, I could tell something big was going down. I called Scott and said, "I think I am going to hold on to this letter for one more day." The next morning I was laid off with a full severance package and two month's salary . . . enough to launch me into my new business. We couldn't believe it, but we should have known. God's economy is always better than ours.

God cares about every part of your life. Your finances included. You are His kid. No matter what financial dilemma you are facing at the moment, you need to know that God loves pulling out all the stops when it comes to providing for you. He is creatively working on your behalf. You may be wondering if you will be able to scrape up enough for rent this month. You may be struggling with the fact that you want to stay home or worrying about who will take care of your little one when you go back to work. Wherever you are, know that He is there. You are not alone. God is not only God of the divine, He is God of the practical. He knows what you need, and the best part is, He can and will take care of you.

Lord,
You care about the smallest details of my life.
I am giving You my worries today.
Thank You for Your daily provision
and Your unending care for me.
I am resting in Your love today.
Amen.

Growing Prayer

Dear heavenly Father,
Thank You for this growing baby who is inside me.
Thank You for shaping his body and molding his soul.
Please grow him strong in Your purpose, Lord.
Strengthen his bones, muscles, organs, and body.
Use Your amazing creativity to form
his hands, feet, arms, and legs.
Please help him to continue to develop at just the right pace
and prepare him to arrive at just the right time.
I commit this precious baby to Your care, Lord.
Thank You for the joy of experiencing growth in a new way.
Amen.

Chapter 12

Little Wonders

THERE ARE SO MANY different things to wonder about when you are pregnant. You wonder if the baby is a he or a she. You wonder what the baby will look like. You wonder if he will arrive on time or stretch out this pregnancy as long as he can. Then you start wondering what kind of person this baby will become . . . will he play basketball, or will he love books? Will she inherit your love of a good dance move, or will she be an adventuress? You wonder what kind of personality this baby will have . . . Will the baby be happy? Colicky? Sleepy? (Let's pray for happy and sleepy!) So. Many. Wonders.

And then there is that wonderful kind of wonder. The wonder of the miracle that you are experiencing. When I was in my second trimester of my first pregnancy, my cousin Beth called to tell me that she was pregnant with her first, too. We just cried on the phone together. Because can there be that much joy? Can the world be that beautiful and lovely? That we would get to experience the joy of being new moms together was too much for us to take in. And that wasn't the only wonder that

I experienced. The whole world seemed brighter to me when I was pregnant (post-nausea, of course). The marvel of all that was taking place inside of me seemed to spill out to everything surrounding the outside of me. Sunsets were exquisite. Coffee dates with friends were mini-celebrations. Life with Scott was rich and good. And there was so much hope for this new life and for our new family. For our new future together. It was all wonder-full. I was seeing a little glimpse of all the wonder that life was meant to hold.

The life your heavenly Father has for you is full of wonder. You are walking out miracle days right now. You, yourself, are full of wonder. Literally. This baby who is growing by leaps and bounds is a testament to God's goodness and love. The intricate processes that are taking place to form his body are too wonder-ful for you to even comprehend. And when you think about it, the very life that you are living, surrounded by the love of family and friends, is a thing of wonder. Can life be this beautiful and lovely? It can. It is. It will be. Bask in the wonder and know that this is only the beginning of all the wonders that God has for you.

Dear Lord,
You are too wonderful for me to comprehend.
I praise You for how You are creating
this baby and for this beautiful world
that You have placed us in.
You are magnificent!
Amen.

My Hopes and Dreams for This Little One

Chapter 13

The Heartbeat

DEPENDING ON how far along you are in your pregnancy, your Ob/Gyn's office may already seem like a second home to you. Your doctors and nurses can become close confidantes . . . but they can also be a little pushy. With ever-increasing regularity, you will find yourself being weighed and measured (not the most fun), being poked and prodded (you won't believe how many tests they come up with), and being questioned about your eating habits and ailments (a little bit like the Spanish Inquisition). But there is one moment during each visit that will bring you a great amount of joy. And that is when your doctor lets you listen to the baby's heartbeat.

Each time my doctor went searching for my baby's heartbeat, I held my breath, as if my not breathing would help her find it quicker. And each time that the *whooshing* sound of my baby's heart filled the room, I would tear up. It was such a good sound. It was the sound of my sweet little one thriving. And when I was in delivery, and they wrapped the heart monitor around my belly so they could track the baby's heartbeat, I loved that, too. I would watch the steady *blip* of the monitor and know that this little one was moments away from being in my arms. Soon I would be able to lay my ear against that little chest and feel the tiny pulse of a heart racing with life. Some moments are too beautiful to describe. That is one of them.

The rhythm of the heartbeat not only brings comfort to you as a mom, but it does to your baby, too. Often, when a new baby is born, he is laid, umbilical cord and all, on the mom's chest so that in that moment of trauma and being brought into all that brightness and light from the dark comfort of the womb, he can once again hear the familiar beat of his mother's heart. Your baby wants to hear the beautiful sound that has sur-rounded him for the past nine months. You and your little one. Your hearts beat for each other.

There is one other heart that beats for you. And that is the heart of your heavenly Father. In that moment of overwhelming love, when you clasp your newborn to your chest, you will get a taste of God's overwhelming love for you. *Who would think you could ever love a little person so much? Who would ever think that God loves you so much?* You can't even begin to understand it. It is too wide and deep and rich for you to comprehend. But know that in those first moments after birth, when you are holding this precious little one close, that God is holding you even closer. Close enough that you can hear His heart.

Lord,
I have experienced Your great love in so many ways.
Help my sweet little one fall
head over heels in love with You.
Draw him in with Your loving-kindness and mercy.
Thank You for the rich life You have given us.
Amen.

Proverbs for the Parent's Heart

He who fears the LORD has a secure fortress,
and for his children it will be a refuge.
Proverbs 14:26

Children's children are a crown to the aged,
and parents are the pride of their children.
Proverbs 17:6

Train a child in the way he should go,
and when he is old he will not turn from it.
Proverbs 22:6

Discipline your son, and he will give you peace;
he will bring delight to your soul.
Proverbs 29:17

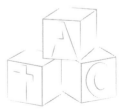

Chapter 14

The Great Feast

YOU MAY BE SURPRISED how hungry you are while you are pregnant . . . especially when the child you are feeding is the size of a peanut. But it is important to remember that you are CREATING an entirely new person within you. That has to take some calories. The pregnant craving is not something to be taken lightly. Baby has some strange ideas about food. (Think potato chip sandwiches and peanut-butter milk shakes.) But I say, go with the cravings. I know I did.

I was determined to eat healthy and not gain a ton of weight with my first pregnancy. But my taste buds were heightened with the onset of baby number one. All of a sudden, my favorite food, chicken, was out. The texture reminded me of a sea slug. Lettuce seemed slimy and disgusting. All I wanted was a cheeseburger. Cheeseburgers are the opposite of healthy eating just in case you didn't know. My plan to nurture my baby with fresh produce was down the toilet. I would get off of work and head straight for the McDonald's drive-through. Scott would get home from work after me and ask, "What's for dinner?" And I would say, "I don't know what you are having, but I had a cheeseburger." It wasn't the best eating plan for our marriage.

Then once I wasn't nauseated anymore, it was if my sense of taste exploded. Food became a feast. Being pregnant seemed to magnify the deliciousness of everything I ate. It was like I was experiencing food in a whole new way. A burrito with green sauce induced tears of joy. Buttered toast with strawberry jam was a delight. Chocolate was something to be adored and reverenced.

Taste wasn't the only sense that was heightened in my life. Pregnancy magnified the beauty of being alive. Once the nausea passed, each day seemed more precious than the last. Getting ready for the baby opened my eyes to the wonderful life God had given me. I was realizing in a new way how very blessed I was. To be embarking on this adventure of having a new family with Scott? I was so thankful. I couldn't contain it.

There is so much goodness to be experienced in this season. Even in the midst of the chaos and weird cravings, you are truly blessed. Let the weight of those blessings rest on you as you move throughout your day. Even when you don't know what is coming around the next bend, you can know this. God is good. And you can dive in to the wide feast of God's goodness. His faithfulness. His grace. His love. He is pouring out His blessings upon you from head to toe, even now. So go on and fill yourself right up.

Lord,

Thanks for this beautiful life You have
given me full of Your goodness,
Your faithfulness, and Your grace.
Continue to pour out Your blessings on this sweet baby.
Amen.

O LORD, you have searched me and you know me.
You know when I sit and when I rise;
you perceive my thoughts from afar.
You discern my going out and my lying down;
you are familiar with all my ways.
Before a word is on my tongue
you know it completely,
O LORD.

—

Psalm 139:1–4

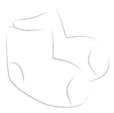

Chapter 15

Oh, Baby!

BABIES ARE the sweetest and cutest people in the world. What is there not to love about them? They are tiny and perfect. With little rosebud mouths and plump cheeks and long eyelashes. And then let's talk about their chubby little arms and legs. So delicious. There is absolutely nothing more precious in this life than a sweet little one. Nothing. There is something so pure and beautiful about newborn babies that it makes our hearts ache with the joy of them.

Scott and I could not help wondering what our first baby would look like. We had seen our nieces and nephews as babies. All adorable. But we had some questions. *Will this baby be chubby or wiry? Fair like Scott or olive-skinned like me? Whose nose would he get? Whose fingers and toes?* We had absolutely no idea what he would look like. We didn't even know if he was a "he." We had decided to wait until delivery to find out if we were having a boy or a girl. We knew we had some good genes going for us. But we also had some weird genes. I was completely bald until I was two. Scott had a blonde afro. What if this baby was bald with tiny patches of blonde afro scattered throughout? Not the best look. What if the baby had Scott's giant head and my giant feet? And that was just the tip of the "What if?" iceberg. On a more sobering note, what if the baby had life-threatening allergies like some of my family members had? What if the baby had more serious physical or mental issues? What if then?

The "what ifs" of pregnancy can lead you to a place of panic because you love this little one so much. But there are always "what ifs" in life. Those "what ifs" are an invitation to trust and lean in to the One who loves you the most of all. It is a hard thing to do. It is hard not to know outcomes. It is hard not to have guarantees. But maybe the question you should be asking is "who?" *Who has given you this baby? Who already knows all the outcomes? Who has crafted this little one with you in mind? Who is shaping your heart to be just the right parent for this little one?* The answer to your "who" question is your heavenly Father. The God of the Universe. So hold off on the panic and run straight into the arms of the One who knows the "whats" and the "ifs." God hears your heart. He wants to flood your soul with His peace and hold you close. And in this moment, His arms are exactly where you need to be.

Lord, I love this little baby growing inside of me.
Breathe Your life and health into him.
I trust You with this little one completely.
Amen.

Sweet Little Bundle of Joy

Sweet little bundle of joy
    Girl or boy
Made up of squeezes and hugs
    Baby bug
How I'm excited, delighted
    Enchanted
Knowing this wonderful wish has been
    Granted

Sweet little ray of sunshine
    Mine all mine
Made up of kisses and stars
    You are ours
How I'm so boisterous and joy-strous and
    Blissing
Knowing that you're the one I'll soon be
    Kissing

Sweet little armful of love
    From above
Made up of laughter and sky
    Lullaby
How I'm enlightened and brightened and
    Glowing

Knowing that you are the reason I'm
Showing

Sweet little hope of my heart
From the start
Made up of blessings and grace
Funny face
Your little life leaps inside me and
Through me
I am so thankful God's giving you
To me.

Chapter 16

So Tired

NOTHING CAN POSSIBLY prepare you for the all-encompassing exhaustion of pregnancy. It feels a little like a nine-month marathon run . . . with a giant stomach. There will be moments in your pregnancy when you would like to lie down and never get up. Even before you start showing, you feel like all of your energy is being rerouted to the baby. Naps are essential. Early bedtimes are a must. If by any chance this is your second pregnancy or third or fourth, then bless your heart. Because the tiredness of pregnancy combined with the tiredness of motherhood is just too much. You may need a year of naps to recover.

When I was pregnant with my first, I went to bed after dinner. I would look at Scott and say, "I think I am ready for bed now." And he would say, "It's 6:30 p.m." And I would say, "Perfect." Finding nap times were a little more difficult during my second and third pregnancies because naps had to coordinate with my kiddos' schedules. I became desperate for my kids to sleep so that I could join them. I don't remember much about those years of my life . . . it is all lost in a haze of sleepiness . . . but we are all alive, so clearly everything turned out as it should.

You may feel like there are not enough hours in the day to get everything done that you want to get done and that napping is the last thing you should be doing. You may feel guilty that you are letting things slide around the house as you burrow beneath the covers for yet another snooze. The fact of the matter is that creating another human inside of your belly is exhausting work. Your body is pulling on every resource to give your baby the nutrition and care that it needs.

In case you were wondering, God is good with naps. After He created the world? He rested. Resting was His idea in the first place. He knows that not only do you need rest physically, but you need it mentally and spiritually, too. Even though there is a lot of excitement and joy in this season, it is also a time of upheaval and change. You need time to nurture your spirit. Your heavenly Father wants to bring your soul to a place of peace and to reenergize you. He cares about your whole person. He wants to rejuvenate you daily. So know that as you rest, God is doing the work in you that you need right now. He is replenishing, reviving, and restoring you, both in body and soul. So relax. Rest in Him and know that He's got you covered.

Lord,
Thank You for the reminder that You offer me rest
both in my body and soul.
You are so good and so generous in
the ways that You love me.
Amen.

Scriptures I Pray Over This Little One

Chapter 17

Pregnancy Pants

THERE IS NOTHING more amazing than seeing the physical evidence of your pregnancy begin to take shape. Your once recognizable belly has begun to reconfigure itself. The first trimester you may not notice a whole lot of belly changes going on. You may be able to slide right into your favorite blue jeans in those first few weeks of blissed-out pregnancy. Then the subtle shift comes. You start to notice a thickening along your waistline. You become a little more solid in your gut. This new little someone is starting to make himself known in a very real way. It is exciting!

And then dawns the day when you realize that, *Sweet Mercy, my pants are really tight.* You have to tug and yank and pull to get them buttoned. Such. Tight. Pants. And the next day? Even tighter. The next week? Forget about it. The time of recognizing the roundness of your belly has arrived. In the interest of keeping your pants on altogether, you need to invest in a good pair of pants made especially for people just like you. People who are growing other people inside of them.

I went the under-the-belly waistband route. I didn't want anything touching my belly. I felt full-fledged over-the-belly maternity panels were restrictive and that if I pulled on them hard enough, I could quite possibly stretch them up over my face like a backward hoodie. But some of my girlfriends wanted the full panel. They felt hugged by the tent-like fabric that shielded their bellies. Do what you need to do. Just find some pants that work for you, that don't cut off your ability to breathe or head south when you bend over to pick up a magazine off of the floor.

You might love this moment of big pants. Or maybe you are struggling with the fact that you gained ten pounds by your first checkup. It is okay to mourn your old pants. And it is also okay to find the best new pants you possibly can for this new belly, this new journey, this new life. Pregnancy is a both/and time of life. Letting go of the old and embracing the new.

Whether this is your first pregnancy or the fifth, your life is shifting on all fronts. God is at work in you doing a new thing. You have never been down this road before. Experiencing these experiences. Feeling these feelings. Embracing a new season can be hard . . . even if it was a season you were looking forward to. Know this. His hand is upon you. His face is turned toward you. He loves you. And He wants to grow you both physically and spiritually, just as He is growing this little one inside your belly. That is a good thing . . . new pants included.

Lord,

I love that You are doing something new in me!
Open my heart to all that You have for me at this time.
I am thankful for Your new mercies every morning.

Amen.

For this reason I kneel before the Father,
from whom his whole family in heaven and
on earth derives its name.
I pray that out of his glorious riches he may
strengthen you with power
through his Spirit in your inner being,
so that Christ may dwell in your hearts through faith.
And I pray that you, being rooted and established in love,
may have power, together with all the saints,
to grasp how wide
and long
and high
and deep
is the love of Christ,
and to know this love that surpasses knowledge—
that you may be filled to the measure of
all the fullness of God.

—

Ephesians 3:14–19

Chapter 18

People Say Weird Things

THERE IS SOMETHING about seeing a pregnant woman that deeply affects people. It breaks down social barriers. It brings smiles to the faces of those all around. Whether you realize or not, you are making a statement each time that you walk into the room. The statement is: *Cutest Baby Ever Coming Soon.* And people are drawn to you. They say things like, "You look amazing!" and "When are you due?" or "Do you know if you are having a boy or a girl?" Everyone wants in on the joy of this new life.

You should know that there will also be weird people who will say mean things to you while you are pregnant. They come out of nowhere and tell you, "You are ENORMOUS! I have never seen anyone so big!" I had a church confrontation once. A lady told me, "I can tell you are having a girl." I said, "You can?" She said, "Yes, because you look pregnant from behind." She might as well have walked up to me and said, "You have a huge rear end." Which, you know, isn't a great thing to say to someone in the best of circumstances.

I bit my tongue. Because she wasn't pregnant and I felt my rear end was decidedly smaller than hers. I think Scott sensed that I was on the brink of saying something irreparable (did I mention he was the youth pastor at this church at the time?). He quickly steered me away from her with soothing words, telling me that, "No one . . . NO ONE . . . can tell you are pregnant from behind and you are beautiful . . . Do you know how beautiful you are? Do you?

These moments when weird people say mean things can break you right down. Or they can make you think violent thoughts about kicking people's kneecaps. The reason it is so upsetting is because you are afraid what they are saying might be true. It is in these moments of hurt (and anger) that you must look past your fears and dig deep to find out what is really true.

The real truth is this: (1) These people are weird. And do you have to believe things weird people say? Nope. You don't. (2) You are beautiful, inside and out, as you grow a whole new person. If growing a baby didn't change your body in some way, you would be the weird one. And the deepest truth of all? (3) You are loved. Deeply. Wholly. Completely. Let the comments and quips roll off of you and know that you are exactly who you are supposed to be right now. God thinks you are the best and most lovely thing He ever created. In fact, He has so much love for you that it cannot be contained. And that is the best truth of all.

Lord,
Thank You for the truth that
I am beautiful and lovable.
Help me to rest in the truth that I am exactly
who I am supposed to be right now.
Thank You for Your deep abiding love every day.
Amen.

Sons are a heritage from the LORD,
children a reward from him.
Like arrows in the hands of a warrior
are sons born in one's youth.
Blessed is the man
whose quiver is full of them.

—

Psalm 127:3–5

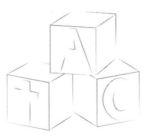

Chapter 19

Weight Watcher

VISITING THE DOCTOR is always an exciting prospect for a new mom. Getting your belly measured and finding out that your baby is growing exactly in the way that she should is amazing. Hearing the baby's heart beat is like witnessing a miracle. Seeing the baby in a sonogram brings home the beautiful reality of this little one who will soon be in your arms. But the practice of having to actually step on the scale yourself at the doctor's office? Not the best. "I wish they would weigh me more. I just can't get enough of it," said no pregnant woman ever.

I went through my first pregnancy in a state of denial. I wouldn't let the nurses tell me how much I weighed. Then came the day when I met with a midwife late in my pregnancy. I told her, "My legs have really been aching when I go walking lately." She laughed and said, "I bet they have. Forty-five pounds is a lot of weight to gain while you are pregnant." I almost passed out. *Forty-five pounds! Sweet Jesus, take me now.* All I could do was laugh with her. The worst had happened. I knew how much I weighed. By my third pregnancy, I had realized something. The scale was going to go up when I got pregnant. And I knew that after I had the baby the scale would go back down. (Maybe not as quickly as I wanted . . .) And the end result? Baby in arms. It was always worth that journey of the scale. ALWAYS.

It's funny how pregnancy can tend to reveal your insecurities and leave you feeling vulnerable and exposed. So many changes are taking place in your heart and soul during pregnancy. Add to that, your body is morphing into a shape you have never seen before, and it is a recipe for feeling out of control. But the truth is that God has created your body in such an amazing way. The morphing? That is all part of the plan. And the fear that your worth is tied to a number on a scale? That is not part of the plan. Let the truth of this season sink into your soul. You are taking part in a miracle. Period. The journey of the scale? It is a part of this season. But it is not the most important part. The most important part is that God has created your body to do an amazing thing—to bring about the arrival of one of the cutest babies ever to grace this earth. It just doesn't get any better than that.

Lord,
Thank You for the perfect gift of this little one joining our family. Help me to let go of the stress and worry of this season and embrace Your goodness. Don't let me lose sight of what is important in this journey. Amen.

Pumpkin Round Baby Sweet

Here we are now just the two of us
    The me of us and now the you of us
        Sitting outside on the park bench singing
            You in my belly round ponging and pinging

I am the brand new mom of you
    Touching and hugging and loving you

Feeling you move as you're stretching and growing
    Rubbing the tummy that you made start showing
        Hearing my voice as I'm laughing and talking
            Feeling me move as I'm dancing and walking

You are my pumpkin round baby sweet
    My safe in my belly round baby sweet

Here we are now just the three of us
    You of us, Dad of us, me of us
        Head on my tummy, he's whispering, giggling
            Loving you, baby, he's feeling you jiggling

He is the brand new dad of you
    Touching and hugging and loving you

Holding me closely, feeling you jumping
    Reading you stories, feeling you bumping
        Dreaming his dreams of you, running and playing
            Filling his mind with you, hoping and praying

You are his pumpkin round baby sweet
    His head near your head round baby sweet

Here we are now just the four of us
    You of us, we of us, Lord of us
        Outside in the garden, laughing and hugging
            Touching the belly, you're kicking and tugging

He is the One who created you
    He shaped you and loved you, created you

He's molding your body small, perfect and growing
    Your personality, happy and glowing
        He knows the soul of you, joyous and pleasing
            He likes to hold you close, loving and squeezing

You are his pumpkin round baby sweet
    His heart near your heart round baby sweet

Here you are now just the one of you
    The perfectly wonderful one of you

Soon we will meet you all brand new and rosy
    Mom and Dad love you from soft head to toes-y

You are the dream and the joy of us
    The sweet little girl or fun boy of us

Full of our happiness, full of our dreaming
    Full of our love and so full of our beaming
        Full of our praying, full of thanksgiving
            Full of our hoping and wishing and living

God bless you pumpkin round baby sweet
    Our wonderful pumpkin round baby sweet

Chapter 20

Belly Buttons

YOU MAY HAVE NOT given much thought to your belly button. Perhaps it has merely served as a decoration for your middle. Maybe it is just something that you strive to keep covered. Whatever you have thought about belly buttons in the past, you might want to take a moment to ponder it. And enjoy it. Before it starts to look and act differently.

Pregnancy does crazy things to belly buttons. Mine flattened out over my round stomach, stretching into a taut line pointing east to west. Some of my friends' belly buttons turned inside out. By the end of their pregnancies, they had popped straight out in a small, round bubble. Everyone's belly button reacts differently. Post-pregnancy, my navel is now shaped more like a frownie face. It has turned down at the corners and folded over on top of itself, as if to say, "I don't care for what you just did to me . . . three times. And now I will show my disdain for you for the rest of your life."

Frownie faces aside, your belly button is important. It is a reminder of your own babyhood and the amazing connectedness that you had to your mom. Belly buttons tell the beginning of your story. In those early, miraculous moments of conception, life began at your belly button level. It was in that exact tiny belly button space that you were completely and wholly connected to your mother. Your lifeline of nutrition and your entire line of defense came to you through your belly button. Your mom shared her immunity, her blood, and her life with you. You had everything you needed to grow and change and become the tiny, perfectly crafted person that you were destined to be.

And now here you are, all these years later, connected to a very tiny person through their belly button. You are sharing your immunity, your blood, and your life with this baby. You are giving them everything that they need to grow and change and become the tiny, perfectly crafted person that they are destined to be. You may have never thought much about your belly button. That is okay. But now you can recognize it for the awe-inspiring thing that it truly is. A point of life-giving connection.

You have a point of life-giving connection with your heavenly Father, too. Your gut-level connectedness is your faith in Him. Your belief that He loves you the most. Your understanding that He can and will sustain you in every circumstance, every messy situation, every vibrant dream, and every mundane day that you face. You can receive every single thing that you need for this life, through Him and in Him. In Him alone, you are truly alive, whole, and growing into the person that He designed you to be. Belly button and all.

Lord,
Remind me that I am only truly alive
when I am connected to You.
I become who You created me to be
when I live in Your presence.
Thank You for Your life-giving Spirit!
Amen.

Good Morning, Baby

As the sun begins to rise
> And the sunbeams warm the air
I feel you moving all around
> Just to let me know you're there.

Did you have good dreams last night
> While you rested safe and sound?
Did you hear the prayers we prayed
> And feel God's angels all around?

Did the beating of my heart
> Gently rock you fast asleep?
Did you hear the lullaby
> That I sang so soft and deep?

Did you hear your Daddy snore
> As he dreamt of holding you?
Did you hear the rain come down
> Or the sprinkle of the dew?

Did the sound of Mommy's laugh
> Wake you from your sleepy dreams?

As I feel you move about
    I stretch and yawn and smile and beam.

Good Morning, little baby mine,
    Welcome to this brand-new day.
Know you're wrapped in Jesus' love
    As you grow and as you play.

Chapter 21

The Pregnant Roller Coaster

UP UNTIL THIS TIME in your life, you may have been a very steady person. You greeted each morning with a great amount of joy and hope. You looked at a problem and found a solution without feeling like it was the end of the world. And then you got pregnant. And your whole emotional state was turned inside out. Your tear ducts have probably not seen this much action in the entirety of your life. You cry whether you are happy, sad, frustrated, or angry. You feel great swells of un-believable happiness followed by horrible lows all in the matter of minutes. Your once rock-solid emotional state is gone . . . welcome to the emotional roller coaster of pregnancy.

When my sister, Erica, got pregnant for the first time, I was in college. I was ecstatic. We were all meeting at my par-ents' house for the weekend, and I had gotten Erica some cute maternity shirts as a surprise. I couldn't wait to show her. As I burst through the door into the bedroom where Erica and her husband, Van, were staying, Erica was sitting on the bed crying and Van was consoling her. I immediately felt sick to my stomach. "What's wrong?" Van looked at me and said, "We don't know." And he looked like he really didn't know. Perplexed. "Do you feel okay?" Erica said, "I'll be okay. Just give me a minute." And she was. A few minutes later, Erica was out in the living room, laughing and doing fine. And I thought, *What in the world was that all about?*

I know now that Erica was riding the pregnancy roller coaster. Almost every pregnant mom experiences this wild ride to some extent. It is as if your normal filter for experiencing and navigating life has been removed and you are feeling everything in the HUGEST WAY POSSIBLE. Happiness. Sadness. Hope. Worry. And it is okay. Really, it is.

When you feel yourself losing it with sorrow or joy or a mix of both, it is exactly the time to remind yourself (1) that you are going to be okay and (2) the One who is completely steady and never changes is on your side. God is not afraid of your hormonal roller coaster. He is not put off by your crazy mood swings and overflow of tears. Spending time in His presence is restorative and calming. He is the One who holds your heart and reminds you, "No matter what you are feeling, I've got you." He knows the outcome of every day. His timing and provision are impeccable. So . . . enjoy the ride.

Lord,
Thank You that even when I am feeling
emotional and freaking out, You aren't.
Thank You for keeping me in a place of safety
and peace and for Your restoring grace.
Amen.

But the fruit of the Spirit is
love,
joy,
peace,
patience,
kindness,
goodness,
faithfulness,
gentleness
and self-control.
Against such things there is no law.

—

Galatians 5:22–23

Chapter 22

The Laying On of Hands

YOU MAY OR MAY NOT be a toucher while you are pregnant. You may love the connection of other people rubbing your belly or you may be more of a "Please keep your hands to yourself" kind of girl. But regardless of what your touchy-feely boundaries are, both you and your baby need some closeness right now. You are made for intimacy. It nurtures your spirit. It lets you know in this time of great change and growth that you are not alone. There is something healing about the touch of another human.

I am somewhat private. Up until pregnancy I had considered my stomach my territory. *If you haven't touched my belly before I became pregnant, you are not invited to touch it while I am pregnant.* The *Touch My Belly* invitation was only given to close friends and family. Of course, some people didn't wait for an invitation. They must have thought, *Well, it's sticking so far out there. Why not?* How about . . . not. I am not the only one who has had their belly touched without an invitation. One of my friends had a strange man she didn't know grab her stomach in the grocery store. I think she should have grabbed his stomach back. You know, just to see how he liked it. That was not the healing connection she was looking for.

While strangers touching me freaked me out, I loved having Scott rest his hand on my belly. That sense of connectedness was exactly what I needed in the more stressful times of my pregnancies. Scott would pray for the baby. Sometimes he would press his hand against my belly and get the baby kicking. And then there were times when he was simply reassuring me that he was with me.

You will need the reassurance of those you love during pregnancy, too. The warm hand of another in yours or a shoulder squeeze. While you absolutely do not need to let your co-worker give you a belly rubdown, you are probably in need of a great deal of hugs from those you love. A good hug is a natural stress reliever. And there is one other touch that you are deeply in need of. That would be God's rich hand of blessing upon your life.

You are daily in need of your heavenly Father's touch. When you are His kid, you get to be the recipient of His calming touch and His healing presence. By His hand, He leads you. He floods your life with peace in your most anxious moments. He is holding you up and holding you close. Now is not the time to pull away from Him. Don't let the craziness of this journey distract you from His nearness. Lean in to Him and His comforting presence. He's got you right in the palm of His hand. And there is no better place to be.

Lord,
Thank You for Your constant presence
in this time of transition.
I trust You to lead me in these coming days.
Thank You again for the blessing of this little one.
Amen.

Fruits of the Spirit Prayer

Dear Holy Spirit,
Thank You for Your presence in this baby's life.
Thank You for the good gifts that You give us.
I ask that You would heap Your blessings upon this little one.
Fill him from head to toe
with Your all-encompassing love and insurmountable joy.
As You mold his spirit,
I pray that You would knead into him Your peace
that passes all understanding.
Grant him patience and goodness as he begins this new life
and grant him the ability to remain faithful to You.
Help him to be gentle to all those around him.
Give him the capacity to control his desires and passions.
Thank You for Your love for this baby.
I commit this precious baby to Your care.
Thank You for Your presence in his life.
Amen.

Chapter 23

It's All About Change

CHANGE IS GOOD. You need change in life to grow and to thrive. If you have not realized it yet, change is what pregnancy is all about. You may have also realized during this great pregnant transition that change is hard. And you may not care if it is good or not. You are probably just thinking, *Let's go back to not changing.*

When I was six months' pregnant with my son, Will, Scott and I moved cross-country from California to Washington, DC. Scott had taken a new job, and we were going to be living with my parents. I was excited about the new adventure we were embarking on. But I felt completely uprooted. All my girlfriends and our church family were back in California. I knew this was exactly where we were supposed to be, but I couldn't seem to get my bearings. I cried. A lot. Scott just looked at me and shook his head and said, "I thought you were happy that we were going to be close to your parents." "I am!" (Said through many tears.) "Then why are you crying?" "I miss my friends. I miss being home." I think Scott also needed to do a lot of deep breathing while I was pregnant. Pregnant women can be a conundrum.

It is funny how when you are going through so many changes in your body that life changes seem to follow. Pregnancy tends to spark all kinds of transition. New jobs. New homes. New friends. The truth is that even though this time of transition can be scary, it can also be one of the best times of your life. Being in that vulnerable state makes you soft and open to new things. Transition is an invitation to become more of the person you were created to be.

It is safe to say that you will not be the same person that you were before you got pregnant. This is hard, but it is good. It is a good time to remember, when everything around you is like shifting sand, that transition is part of God's plan. His plan has always been about transformation. He wants you to be open to all of the goodness that He has for you in this season. He wants you to know that you don't have to make all these changes on your own. His plan is that you rely completely on Him. He wants to fortify you with His love and build you up with His peace. And that is a truly beautiful thing, too.

Lord,
You are the Master Planner.
I can see even in these last months of pregnancy
how You are weaving my life together.
Thank You for shaping me and changing me
and growing me in new ways.
Amen.

Safe in Your Arms Prayer

Dear Jesus,
Thank You for this small person growing inside of me.
Thank You for the miracle that is happening,
moment by moment, inside of my body.
I am so glad that You know this baby inside and out.
I am so glad that You care for him even more than I do.
Please wrap Your arms of love and protection
around this tiny baby.
Please keep this wee one safe in Your arms
as he grows in my body.
I commit this precious baby to Your care.
Thank You for Your gift of life in this new little baby.
Amen.

Chapter 24

The Love Lens

ONCE YOU ARE PREGNANT, you see the whole world through a baby-tinted lens. It is bright and rosy and new. And it should be. This is a wonderful time of your life. You are immersing yourself in all things baby. Pregnancy websites. Baby magazines. Baby boutiques. Prenatal workouts. These are the things that interest you. This is completely normal. Because once you are pregnant, your entire outlook on life is transformed. This baby is revolutionizing the way that you live and see life.

When I got pregnant, I developed a kind of pregnant radar. Everywhere I looked, there were pregnant people and babies of all ages and strollers and more pregnant people. It seemed like the whole world was pregnant. I know this is not true, but it seemed true. My eyes had been opened to the world of babies. And suddenly everything that was important to me had to do with this wonderful new addition in my life.

Don't be surprised if the baby lens starts to change what is most important to you, too. Your desires can change. Your dreams and hopes can change. Even your fears can change. One pregnant friend said that she could no longer watch the news.

Any time a sad story would come on she would think, *That is someone's baby,* and burst into tears. It is not that she hadn't cared about the news before, but her frame of reference was shifting. She was becoming a different person altogether. She was looking at life through the lens of a mom's love. She wanted to protect, hold, and keep safe all the babies of the world.

Your heavenly Father also has a love lens. Just as you can't stop thinking about your baby, He can't stop thinking about you. Isn't that a crazy thought? He cannot get His mind off of you. It says in the Psalms that He delights in the details of our lives. Everything He has done in the past and is doing now is for the love of His precious kids. His love for you shapes your life and destiny. He wants to protect, hold, and keep safe all the babies of the world. That includes your baby. That includes you. When you get a little taste of that amazing love, you can only have one response . . . loving Him back with everything that is in you. And if you think about it . . . the best lens of life that you can ever have is the one where you are wrapped up in His love, loving Him back.

Lord,
I want to love You with all my heart, with all my soul, with all my mind, and with all my strength. May this little one have that same heart cry. Thank You for loving us first. Amen.

The LORD your God is with you,
he is mighty to save.
He will take great delight in you,
he will quiet you with his love,
he will rejoice over you with singing.

—

Zephaniah 3:17

Chapter 25

The Fullness of Joy

THE PREGNANT BELLY is a marvel to behold. Who in the world could think that you could fit another person into your body? As far as you knew, you had just enough room for all your own parts and innards. And now here you are, experiencing the daily miracle of a growing baby inside of you. And in a perfect kind of way, your organs shift, your rib cage expands, your pelvis widens. Room is made to accommodate this incredible life inside of you. Some room anyway. You may be finding as the months progress that this little love can wedge a sharp elbow or a tiny foot under your rib cage. His favorite place to take his morning nap could quite possibly be sitting on your bladder. You may also find that you need to stand up to get in a good deep breath. Your lungs need to find a way to expand around all that baby.

The upside of being full of baby is that you can almost start identifying his body parts as he tucks and rolls inside of you. You will find yourself saying, "That's a foot!" "Here is his tush!" And "Is that his head?" Depending on how tall you are, you may reach your fullness point earlier on than your pregnant girlfriends. My cousin, Beth, is five feet tall. Early on in her pregnancy she realized, "Houston, we have a problem." There was a whole lot of baby and not a whole lot of Beth. She had to do a lot of stretching and maneuvering to get comfortable. There will come a moment when you, too, realize, "You know what, kid? There is just not enough room in this body for the both of us." And that is the goal. It's not a bad thing. You are full up to the top with new life. You have done exactly what you were supposed to do. You have grown this baby so that he can join you in the world.

In so many ways, your heavenly Father is in on this sense of fullness. He is filling you up to the top with grace as you navigate these last few weeks of pregnancy. He is filling you up with hope at the thought of bringing new life into the world. And He is, even now, giving you all the strength and stamina that you need, even when you can't seem to get a full breath. So enjoy every moment of being full. Let the fullness overwhelm you. And know that someday soon, all that love, hope, and joy filling you up will be a beautiful bundle of baby in your arms.

Lord,
Every morning that I wake up and feel this little one
growing inside of me, I sense Your presence.
Your joy has filled me to overflowing.
Thank You for Your gift of new life.
Amen.

Tender Heart Prayer

Lord Jesus,
Thank You for Your gift of eternal life.
I pray that even as this baby is inside of me,
You will begin to draw his heart close to You.
Please give him Your heart of compassion and tenderness.
Prepare his heart to hear how You came to save us
from ourselves and to know deep inside that
You are good and right.
Help him to accept Your gift of salvation at a young age.
Please help him to grow each year in his knowledge
of Your love for him and for those around him.
Please show him how to come to You even when he is afraid
and ashamed of the things that he has done wrong.
Hold him close to You as he walks on his life's journey
and don't ever let him go.
I commit this precious baby to Your care, Jesus.
Thank You for revealing Yourself to us so that
we could know You forever.
Amen.

Chapter 26

Songs of Delight

TALKING TO YOUR BELLY is a normal practice during pregnancy. You will regularly see pregnant moms chatting it up with their babies. "What are you doing in there?" "Wow . . . you are busy today." And, "Could you please remove your knee from my kidney?" These are all regular conversations. But talking with your baby isn't the only way that you can connect. What is really fun is playing your favorite music for your belly. If you are a hard-core country music fan, you might as well start training up your little cowboy now. If you are convinced that your sweet girl could quite possibly be a ballerina, because of all of her leaps and turns, why not foster her dance moves with a little "Dance of the Sugar Plum Fairy"? Music is the language of the soul.

Some of my friends put headphones on their bellies to pipe in their favorite tunes. One of my friends played the piano and sang to her belly. Another friend's husband strummed the guitar and serenaded her babies regularly. My husband, Scott, would rap to our babies. He wanted them to be well rounded musically.

I sang to my babies in utero. When I would rock my two-year-old, Will, to sleep for his afternoon nap, I sang to my belly, too. I wanted Addison to hear my voice. I had one arm around Will and one hand on my belly. I wanted Addie to sense my love. I wanted him to connect the sound he was hearing with the person who loved him and cherished him completely. Somehow my lullabies always turned into worship songs. I would begin to sing about God's love and His mercy. And how much He loved these little ones—both the one on my lap and the one in my belly. And I don't think that I was the only one singing.

God sings songs of delight over His kids constantly. He is just like you when you are crooning to your little one. Or maybe it is more that you are just like Him. He finds a great deal of delight in you and who He has created you to be. He wants to reassure you with His constant love and faithfulness. When you are talking to your baby and singing songs of love to her, you are the mirror image of your heavenly Father. So with a loving hand on your belly, talk and sing and play music to your heart's content and know that He is joining in with your song.

Lord,
I love the thought of You taking delight in me
and this little one.
Thank You for filling us to overflowing with Your love,
singing us lullabies and love songs.
We adore You.
Amen.

Songs That I Sing and Play for This Baby

1. _____
2. _____
3. _____
4. _____
5. _____
6. _____
7. _____
8. _____
9. _____
10. _____
11. _____
12. _____
13. _____
14. _____
15. _____
16. _____
17. _____
18. _____
19. _____
20. _____

Chapter 27

Baby Gymnastics

THERE IS NOTHING more fantastic than lying down with both hands on your pregnant belly and feeling the fluttering kicks of a teeny, tiny human pummeling the underside of your hands. They are love kicks. Maybe they are not even kicks. Maybe they are full-body love somersaults. Or love push-ups. Who knows? What you know is that it is a beautiful feeling.

When I was pregnant with my second son, Will, I knew that I would have a very active baby on my hands. The child simply would not stay still. When I lay down, he took it as his cue for a gymnastics routine. He used my innards as a jumping-off place for his acrobatics. He would lodge a small foot near the back of my left bottom rib and launch himself into a series of dolphin-like moves. By my third trimester, the show was quite impressive. Better than TV. The ripples of my belly looked like the rolling waves of the ocean. It was our nightly entertainment, seeing how many weird shapes my stomach could take on. Oval. Circle. Trapezoid? Wherever he kicked, I would press back, letting him know I loved feeling him move.

When my sister, Jenny, was visiting from her work overseas in Africa, she wanted to get in on the action. She had heard how wild Will would get at night, and she wanted to see it for herself. I lay back on my bed. Within seconds, he was tucking and rolling. We couldn't stop laughing. Jenny put her cheek against my rolling stomach and said, "I love you, Baby Will." He thumped back against her cheek. She popped up. "He kicked me! He heard me!" That little kick was Will's hello. He wanted to connect with that person talking to him. His Creator formed him that way.

When you press up against that hard ball of baby in your belly, you are connecting with your little one, saying hello. You are letting her know that you see her and feel her and love her. She was made to connect with you. It is how her Creator formed her. It is how your Creator formed you, too.

In these days of high joy and hormones, your Creator is still looking for that connection with you, His daughter. Are you aware of how much He is reaching out to touch your heart on a daily basis? With beauty. With nature. With those around you. With His Word. With the whispers of His Holy Spirit to your mommy's heart. He is a hands-on kind of heavenly Father looking for connectedness with you. You may not have ever thought about God wanting to connect with you. He longs to know you in every way and to flood your life with His grace and mercy. And when you think about it, that is the most beautiful thing of all.

Lord,
I love that You want to connect with me.
I want to be connected to You.
Bring me close to You.
Thank You for Your great goodness!
Amen.

And whoever welcomes a little child
like this in my name welcomes me.

—

Matthew 18:5

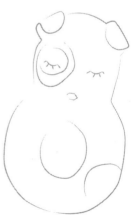

Chapter 28

The Name Game

THERE IS NOTHING more fun than picking out a name for your baby. So many books, websites, and baby magazines are dedicated to the art of naming your precious little one, you can spend hours perusing them. You have just under a gazillion names to choose from. There are so many adorable names out there. And a whole lot of weird ones. You want to get this right. You don't want your child coming to you, asking, "Really? What in the world were you thinking giving me this name?" So, no pressure, Mom . . . take all the time you want picking it out. Your child will just be carrying it around for the rest of her life.

I have always loved the name Jack. It is such a good, strong name. My husband, Scott, liked it, but he was more adamant about what we would name our first baby if we had a girl. He wanted to name her Destiny. Destiny. I asked him, "Are we hippies now?" He said, "No. But years from now when she brings home a boy who wants to date her, I want to be able to say, 'She's not your Destiny.'" "You can't name our child a name just because of something that you want to say to her future boyfriend." Scott disagreed. He wanted Destiny. So we made a deal. If the baby was a boy, it would be Jack. If it was a girl, it would be Destiny. Jack is super glad he was a boy.

Middle names can be difficult, too. One syllable? Two syllables? Does it go well together with your last name? And what about the meaning? You don't want to name your child something that has a horrible meaning. Jack's middle name is Riley, which means "valiant." I overheard him telling one his friends, "Ya . . . my middle name is Riley . . . I think it means violent." We are going to have to work on that. I didn't do much better with girl's names. If Will had been a girl, I wanted to name her "Sophie Kate." Until my niece pointed out that that name combo sounded a whole lot like "suffocate." Not so good. Tread carefully in the choosing of names. You don't want to choose something you will regret.

There is one fantastic name that has already been given to your baby. The moment your baby was conceived, your heavenly Father stamped her with His family name. She is marked with His love. She is crafted by His hand. She is made in His image. And her name has been engraved in His palm. She is completely known by the One who put the stars in the sky. She is beloved by the One who commands the sea and directs the winds. It may be too wonderful for you to comprehend, but the One with the Name above all names has a way with words. And He is calling your little one . . . child of God. That is the best name of all.

Lord,

Thank You for naming this baby as one of
Your children and creating her in Your image.
May her heart be like Yours, too,
filled with love and peace.
Bless this little one today.
Amen.

Baby Names That I Love

(boys) (girls)

1. _____	1. _____
2. _____	2. _____
3. _____	3. _____
4. _____	4. _____
5. _____	5. _____
6. _____	6. _____
7. _____	7. _____
8. _____	8. _____
9. _____	9. _____
10. _____	10. _____
11. _____	11. _____
12. _____	12. _____
13. _____	13. _____
14. _____	14. _____
15. _____	15. _____
16. _____	16. _____
17. _____	17. _____
18. _____	18. _____
19. _____	19. _____
20. _____	20. _____

Chapter 29

The Best Nest

NESTING IS A THING. Just in case you have never been pregnant before and you were thinking it wasn't. Maybe you don't even know what nesting is. Just imagine a sweet mama bird, carrying little twigs to its nest, fiddling with feathers, weaving little puffs of cotton and twine into her new home, getting everything ready for the new little eggs that she will lay any day now. Now imagine that mama bird is a large, highly motivated pregnant woman with an entire house to re-organize before the baby arrives, and you have some idea of what nesting is.

Scott came home from work one day to find our entire living room rearranged. I was eight months' pregnant at the time. He looked around and said, "What happened? Who moved all the furniture around?" I grinned and said, "I did." Then he got upset. "Sue! That isn't safe for you or the baby. You are not supposed to lift anything!" "I didn't!" "Then how did you move all the furniture?" "With my rear." "With your what?" "My rear . . . I leaned on everything and pushed it into place." Then Scott just looked scared. Because I had become an irrational person who rearranged entire rooms on a whim with my rear. The nesting instinct could not be denied.

There is something very sacred about nesting. A little bit of heaven is about to come to earth in the form of a sweet baby. Nesting is your response. In each little nesting act, a piece of your mother's heart is revealed. You want your baby to be safe. You want his surroundings to be welcoming. You want him to know that he is cared for and loved. Underneath all of your obsessive-compulsive cleaning impulses beats the heart of a mama who is beside herself with joy at the prospect of mothering this little one. You simply cannot hold it in. Your heart beats for this baby. Every room in the house shows it. You want this baby to know you've got him covered in every possible way.

This nesting process mirrors the Father heart of God for you. All this care, all this love that you have, reflect how God has set up the world around you. The path of hope that He has you on. The blessings that He has poured out on you over and over again. He wants you to be safe. He wants you to know that you are loved and cared for. He is the ultimate Caretaker. He cares for you, body, mind and spirit. So take a moment to recognize all of that loving-kindness coming your way and relax. He's got you covered . . . in every possible way.

Lord,
You are my refuge, and I take shelter in
the shadow of Your wings.
You are faithful in every way.
Thank You for Your daily provision
and for Your covering.
Amen.

The LORD bless you and keep you;
the LORD make his face shine upon you
and be gracious to you;
the LORD turn his face toward you
and give you peace.

—

Numbers 6:24–26

Chapter 30

What You Really Need

AS YOU ARE GETTING your house, your car, and your life ready to accommodate a new baby, it is very hard to determine the difference between wants and needs. What do you really need for this new baby? Clothes. Blankets. A crib. A car seat. A baby bath. Then there are the wants that feel like needs. Adorable bedding for the crib. Stylish nursery décor. An abundance of baby outfits. You want everything to be just right when this little baby comes. Most pregnant mommies do. As a brand-new mom, you may not be sure what you really need, so you feel like you need everything . . . just in case. Oh . . . and everything needs to be cute, of course.

Our baby budget was never very big. Scott and I couldn't deck out a new nursery for each baby. But with each pregnancy, God seemed to go out of His way to provide exactly what we needed through friends, co-workers, and family. What I truly needed? I had. A loaned wicker bassinet for Jack. A new car seat for Will. And some of the deepest unspoken wants that I thought might be frivolous? Somehow those found their way into my nursery, as well. When my sisters and cousin Beth found out there was a set of crib bedding I wanted for my third, Addison, they surprised me with it. When I opened it, I cried. It seemed as if God was letting me know, "I see you. I even know these little hidden wants that you have." It might not seem like a big deal. But to me it was a huge deal. It was as if His hand of blessing was upon me, in a physical way. Not only was He providing for us practically, but He was providing for me on a very real and personal level. He saw the secret desires of my heart and provided for those, too.

It is not wrong for you to want to care and provide for this baby in the best way possible. That is exactly what your heavenly Father wants to do for you, too. God has promised to provide you with every single thing that you need. He sees you and He knows you. He has been planning for this baby's arrival. He knows the desires of your heart, and He knows what this little one needs. You can relax and know that He will take care of you and this baby. And He will surprise you in the practical and loving ways that He does so. He is generous, and His kindness will enfold you. You can count on it.

Lord,
Thank You for supplying my every need.
And thank You for surprising me with Your blessings.
You give me more than I want and need in so many ways.
You are always enough for me.
Amen.

In the morning, O LORD, you hear my voice;
in the morning I lay my requests before you
and wait in expectation.

—

Psalm 5:3

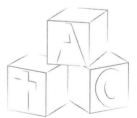

Chapter 31

Help Is on the Way

THE LONGER THAT YOU ARE pregnant, the more help you will need to function throughout the day. The physical demands of carrying a large amount of weight out in front of you can start to take its toll. The labor part of pregnancy seems to start long before your contractions set in. Getting in and out of bed may require some assistance. Tying your shoes is no small thing. You may be able to reach your feet, but the act of bending down can cut off all air supply. Shoes start to seem less important. You will notice that some of your pregnant friends opt for flip-flops at this point. Don't do it. You will regret it.

I speak from experience. One Sunday late in my first pregnancy, I tried to slip out of church during the service. The edge of my flip-flop caught on the carpet, and I tripped as I exited my row. Our entire church saw me hurtling down the aisle. The congregation gave a collective gasp. I grabbed for the first person I could. I found myself on my knees, gripping a very surprised visitor. She gripped me back. From the pulpit, our pastor (who had stopped speaking at the time of my launching) asked, "Are you okay?" As I got to my feet, I said loudly for all to hear, "I'm okay," and to the visitor, "Thanks for catching me." I needed all the help I could get.

You will need all kinds of help in the weeks before you give birth. You will need help carrying out your groceries. You will need people to pick up things for you off of the floor. And you will need to know this. Needing help is not a sign of weakness. It is a sign of strength. You are recognizing your limitations and asking others to bridge the gap for you. This is not being selfish. It is necessary. And the people who love you the most are happy to bridge that gap. They want to help you.

Your heavenly Father has always wanted to bridge the gap of your weakness with His strength. It is His promise to you. In your weakness, He is strong. What you lack? He has in spades. What you need? He can provide. Needing help while you are pregnant is just a part of this season. But needing God's help? That is a part of life from now until you see Him in eternity. He is your ever-present help in times of trouble. He is your refuge. Your shelter. Your strong tower. He will never leave you or forsake you. No matter what season of life, pregnant or not . . . you can always come to Him for help.

Lord,
You are the One who keeps me safe.
Thank You for always catching me.
Thank You for Your amazing faithfulness.
Amen.

Blessings for Baby

Write a prayer of blessing for your baby.

Chapter 32

Generations

THIS SWEET BABY in your belly is forming a new little branch on your family tree. A new generation is being launched. This is a new addition to the long line of babies that God has created in your family. You may be praying that there are certain family traits that He includes when He is forming your little one. (Grandma June had the sweetest disposition.) And . . . you may be hoping that there are certain family traits that He leaves out when He is forming your little one. (Great-Uncle Larry is out of control.) But mostly, you are praying and hoping that this little one, no matter what his future successes and struggles, knows Jesus and His great love.

When I was pregnant with my second son, Will, I was asked to sing Sara Groves's song, "Generations," for our church's three services on Mother's Day. Sara is one of my favorite songwriters in the world. I was honored to sing her poignant lyrics about how the choices we make affect the ones we love most of all. Our children. And our children's children. And every time I got to the place in the song where she speaks out a life of peace over her great-great-great-grandchildren, my eyes would well up with tears. Because it was such a good thing to speak out. Such a huge hope and a huge prayer for those who come along behind us.

When I was singing the song, I was singing for my boys. I was hoping especially that the blessing of peace in the song would start with Will and Jack. That their sweet little lives would be blanketed in the peace of the One who loves them most of all. And that the trickle-down effect of my choices, of Scott's choices, and of our babies' choices, would rain down on every branch of our family tree. It was and still is my great hope, that we would all be rooted in the love of Christ . . . generation after generation. Living in hope. Living in peace.

Praying for peace over your baby is a good thing to do. But it is more than that. It is a powerful thing to do. Just as your choices can affect the generations that come behind you? Your prayers carry the weight of blessing with them down through the generations. When you pray for your baby, it will bless your grandkids. Isn't that a crazy thought? And isn't that a beautiful thought? Your heavenly Father's greatest desire is to be close to you . . . and to your children . . . and to your grandchildren. When you take a moment to pray a blessing of peace over your baby, you are shifting things in the heavenlies. God will move heaven and earth to keep your baby close to His heart. So start saying the prayers now that will shape your family tree for generations to come, rooting them in the love of Jesus. There is nothing more powerful than that.

Lord,
Thank You for the blessing of family.
May the blessings of our good choices
pour out over this baby.
May she live in peace and hope to the end
of her days and pass on that legacy
to her own children and grandchildren.
Amen.

How priceless is your unfailing love!
Both high and low among men find refuge
in the shadow of your wings.
They feast on the abundance of your house;
you give them drink from your river of delights.
For with you is the fountain of life;
in your light we see light.
Continue your love to those who know you,
your righteousness to the upright in heart.

—

Psalm 36:7–10

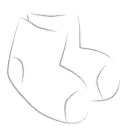

Chapter 33

Resting Up

HAVE YOU EVER TRIED to rest with an eight-pound medicine ball tied to your stomach? Or tried to get some REM sleep while getting up three times an hour to use the restroom? No? Well, welcome to your last few weeks of pregnancy. Do what you must to get in some precious moments of sleep. You are going to need them.

I remember Scott eyeing the bed one night after I had arranged myself to go to sleep. I had two pillows under my head. One pillow between my knees. One pillow behind my back and one pillow propping up my giant stomach. He said, "I'm not sure there is actually room in there for me." I was wedged in. I grinned up at him. "Sorry . . . it's the only way I can sleep."

He shook his head at the sorry state of our marriage. I think he expected more from me. Maybe a little "I can't wait to snuggle with you . . . we can work this out." I didn't offer condolences. This was how it was going to go down. Because sleep is like gold. Precious. You must cling to it. He said something like, "You've changed, Sue," then he smiled and kissed my forehead. He grabbed the one unused pillow and headed for the couch. Scott knew what I needed. A good night's sleep and 400 pillows. That made me fall in love with him even more.

Scott knew that I was trying to store up energy for the coming days. I was cocooning myself in blankets and pillows, soaking up the last moments of uninterrupted sleep before I embarked on one of the hugest transitions in my life . . . new mommy-hood. I knew it was going to take all that I had to give and then some. I wanted to be ready for all the beauty, joy . . . and sleepless nights that were headed my way.

In these last weeks before you meet your baby, you may be feeling the same way. As you get ready to launch into this new phase of life, it is a good thing to rest up. It is a good thing to know your limits and to shore up your strength. And it is an especially good thing to know that your heavenly Father is paving the way for you. Like being surrounded with fluffy pillows, He is hemming you in on every side with His mercy and grace. He knows that you are tired and anxious. He knows what you need. He wants you to know that He will be with you every step of the way. So grab your pillows and snuggle in . . . He is holding you in His arms and great joy is just around the corner.

Lord,
You are with me every moment of every day.
Thank You for surrounding me on every side
as I get ready for this huge adventure of motherhood.
I am thankful for Your knowledge
of me and care for me.
Amen.

Mom and Baby Fun Facts

The day I found out I was pregnant with you was _____

When I read the pregnancy test, I said _____

When I told Daddy you were coming, he said _____

We had our first prenatal checkup on _____ with

    Doctor _____

The food I crave the most is _____

The smell I can't stand is _____

The first thing I bought for you was _____

The first day I wore maternity pants was _____

The first time I felt you kick was _____

The first time Daddy felt you kick was _____

Your favorite time of day to move is _____

Your favorite time of day to be still is _____

Your number in the grandkid lineup is _____

Your number in our family lineup is _____

My favorite baby magazine is _____

My favorite baby website is _____

My favorite song to play for you is _____

My favorite book to read to you is _____

I know I am nesting and getting ready for you because _____

_____

The nickname Daddy and I call you is _____

Chapter 34

Birthing People

THE CLOSER YOU GET to your delivery date, the more you start thinking about two things: (1) This baby has to come out NOW! and (2) This baby has to come out HOW? You are definitely ready to be done with pregnancy. With the swollen legs and the sleepless nights. And those Braxton Hicks contractions that pull your entire belly into a hard round ball? Those you could do without. But the reality of the way that this baby is going to have to exit your body? It is off-putting to say the least.

The week before I delivered my first son, Jack, I looked at Scott and said, "You have the hugest head I have ever seen." He said it is one of the more hurtful things that I have ever said to him. But I had suddenly realized, *Hey! This baby could have a giant head. That is not good.* I wasn't talking about it a whole lot. But I was freaked out. Birthing a person, no matter how big or small, was something I had never done before. My prayer became, "Sweet Jesus! Help this kid have a small head." Is that an okay prayer to pray? I think so. But I think I started praying it too late. All three of my boys inherited their Dad's large dome. ALL THREE. No thank you.

Childbirth is one of those things where pain comes with the territory. You should know that quite a few of us moms are super thankful for drugs . . . we also have a great fondness for anesthesiologists. You should also know that I have yet to meet a mom who said, "I love the pain of childbirth." That would be weird. But every mom I have met said, "It was completely worth it!"

When I look back on the deliveries of my boys, it is not that it didn't hurt . . . it is that it didn't matter. In light of the joy that was delivered, I just didn't care. I was over the moon with the love of them. I couldn't get enough of those babies. Miracles, every one. All I had to do was put my face near that sweet little (GIANT) head of my son and think, *Oh my Lord, I would do it all again a million times over.* It was worth it. So worth it.

Pain was a part of the love process for your heavenly Father, too. The enormous sacrifice? Giving His Son up for you? Feeling the pain of loss and separation? He did it all for that beautiful moment of reconciliation. That moment when you were restored to His arms and He could hold you close. He is over the moon with the love of you. He can't get enough of you. He thought it was worth it. He thought you were worth it. And aren't you are so glad that He did?

Lord,
Thank You for all that You
went through on my behalf.
I can feel Your love surrounding me
and know that You are holding me close.
Thank You for giving up Your Son
so that I could have new life in You.
Amen.

Hello Baby

Hello Baby, Hello Light
Hello Precious, Hello Bright
You are mommy's bumblebee
Her quite delicious cup of tea.

At this moment in this place
I can't wait to see your face
Kiss your fingers, kiss your nose
Kiss your elbows, kiss your toes
I just want to squeeze you tight.
My love for you is day and night.

Hello Cutie, Hello Sweet
Hello Sunshine, Hello Treat
You are daddy's happy tune
His taste of sun and slice of moon.

At this moment, all the while
He can't wait to see your smile
Hear your giggle, soothe your cry
Join your laughter, feel your sigh
He just wants to sing with glee.
His love for you is sky and sea.

Hello Honey, Hello Love
Hello Sweet Pea, Hello Dove
You are Jesus' very own
His joy, His heart, His child, His poem.

At this moment, from the start
He can't wait to fill your heart
Sense your spirit, hear your thoughts
Touch your soul and love you lots.
He just wants to twirl and leap.
His love for you is wide and deep.

At this moment, where you are
Of all the babies near and far
We're so thankful that you're ours
Full of hopes and dreams and stars
We can't wait until your birth.
Our love for you is heav'n and earth.

Chapter 35

All the Waiting

YOU ARE PROBABLY much better at waiting than I am. You might be filled to brimming with patience and long-suffering. You are most likely kind and gentle and full of grace in every kind of waiting circumstance. It could be that you are a much better person than I am in general.

I could have done without all the waiting during pregnancy. Waiting to find out if I was actually pregnant. Waiting for morning sickness to be done. Waiting for doctor visits. Waiting for test results. Waiting for maternity leave. And then there was the ultimate waiting . . . waiting for the baby to actually come. Patience does not come naturally to me. I am really so much better at being impatient. I have years of practice under my belt.

When I went to my due-date checkup with my firstborn, the doctor said, "Well, that is amazing. That baby still has a ton of room and your amniotic fluid looks like you could even go for another couple of weeks." I lay on the table and furiously blinked back tears. This baby was supposed to be due. He was not supposed to hang out in my belly for two more weeks.

Doesn't he know how tight my pants are? Doesn't he understand that I can no longer breathe when I sit down? I was through. All I wanted was to be done. But much like most babies, Jack did not care. I could be through all I wanted. He was going to stay put until the perfect moment, when it was his time to make his entrance. He was in God's hands. My timetable had very little to do with it. I could have done with less anger and more hope.

Hope is exactly what you need in these hours . . . days . . . weeks of waiting. Focusing on the wait can get you tense and uptight and maybe even a little angry. But with hope, you get to rely on your heavenly Father for His timing, His plan, His path for you in this moment. With hope, you get to focus on the beauty of what is to come. All that love and grace and mercy poured out when that sweet little baby is nestled in your arms. So take that deep breath. Know that in exactly the right moment in time, your wait will be over. And know that just as you are hoping for that moment of feeling that little one in your arms, your heavenly Father has you wrapped in His.

Lord,
All of my hopes and dreams for this baby,
I give back to You. I know that You will bring him
in exactly the right time. Thank You for the good gift
of this precious little one.
Amen.

*I prayed for this child, and the LORD
has granted me what I asked of him.*

—

1 Samuel 1:27

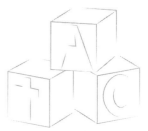

Chapter 36

So Huge

YOU COULD COMPARE your pregnancy experience to that of a butterfly. There is that beautiful, life-altering change that happens when you graduate from woman to mother. You are transformed with a love so deep and true that you will never be the same again. Unfortunately, your capacity to love is not the only thing that has grown by leaps and bounds. There is a certain point in pregnancy where most things start to take on giant proportions. Your excitement. Your joy. And your stomach. All huge.

For me, the most drastic huge-ness came with my third pregnancy. I had gone to see my doctor for my 38-week check-up. As I lay back on the exam table, I could barely see over my stomach as she leaned over to measure it. She glanced over at my chart and then back at me. "You know, last week you were measuring 37 weeks (perfect), but this week you are measuring 40 weeks (ginormous)." I sat up on the table. "That is what I was saying to you. Do you see this?" I said, pointing to the bulging sides of my stomach. "My stomach has never looked like this. It is growing sideways now." She nodded. "Yes, I see this. I am thinking we can't let this baby go until your due date. We may have to induce."

And I was thinking, *Yes, dear God, please induce right now!* Because both of my other babies had been nine pounds. *How giant is this child going to be? How much longer can we let this kid go?* He was trying to bust out my sides. As it happened, Addison came five days early without induction. As they laid him on my chest and I wept tears of joy, I also had the thought, *Hey, this baby is not small.* He was nine pounds, twelve ounces. I had birthed a linebacker. A really super-sweet, adorable linebacker.

There are so many things during pregnancy that seem huge—your stomach being only one of them. Your worries can be huge. Your physical ailments can be huge. Your responsibilities can be huge. But the thing that you don't want to forget is the hugeness of your heavenly Father's grace. So. Much. Grace. Grace upon grace upon grace meets you around every corner. Huge grace for your anxious thoughts. Huge grace for your struggles—whether they are physical, financial, or emotional. There is no situation or moment that you are going to experience that cannot and will not be met with the supply of God's unending grace. Even the moment when you realize your baby might be enormous. There is grace for that, too. So let it roll over you, surround you, and lift you as you realize His grace is enough to meet your every need. Because realizing that . . . is huge.

Lord,

Thank You for the hugeness of Your grace.

It is enough for me in every situation.

You are so good to me.

Amen.

Trust in the LORD with all your heart
and lean not on your own understanding;
in all your ways acknowledge to him
and he will make your paths straight.

—

Proverbs 3:5–6

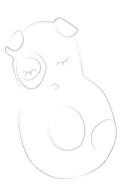

Chapter 37

The Big Squeeze

ONE OF THE BIGGEST UNKNOWNS in pregnancy is trying to figure out if you are actually having a baby. Are the contractions you are feeling just Braxton Hicks? Should you lounge around your house for another couple of days, or will you birth someone in the car if you don't leave for the hospital right now? There is one thing you may have figured out as you start feeling the tightening of your gut. Contractions are not the most comfortable thing in the world. Anyone who tells you differently probably hasn't experienced them.

I made Scott take me to the hospital. Twice. Only to have the nurses tell me, "No, you are not in labor. Go back home." I asked them several times, "Are you sure I am not in labor? These things hurt." They just smiled and said, "We can give you some medication so you can rest, but you are not in labor." I said, "No . . . I will be okay." And then Scott drove me home, and I lay awake for five more hours having "fake" contractions. I should have taken the drugs: (1) because I'm not a fan of pain, and (2) because I was scared. If these weren't real contractions, then what in the world were real contractions going to be like?

I found out. When real labor hit, my birth plan of walking around and sitting on a labor ball flew straight out the window. I had this brilliant thought, *I think I am going to just lie down . . . until they hand me a baby.* I did my breathing exercises. I held Scott's hand. I nibbled on ice chips. I requested drugs. And I labored. This baby was putting the squeeze on me. But the biggest surprise was that the all-consuming fear of the dreaded contractions had slipped away. Because I was doing it. I was making it. I was having real contractions. In the midst of the big squeeze, I had a new focus. All that mattered was seeing that baby.

Labor isn't the only time in life when you will feel the squeeze of pain in your life. But our heavenly Father always has a plan for the difficulties you are walking through. The end goal of labor is a baby. But the end goal of God working in your life is for you to be like Him and to have His mind and heart. No one likes pain. But He never lets you go through anything alone. Whatever big squeezes you encounter in life? He has something good to bring from it. He wants to give you a new focus. That focus is Him. Keep your heart focused on His love, His grace, and His goodness. And He will birth something beautiful and new in your life.

Lord,

I don't like pain, but I know that You can bring
beauty out of the most difficult things in my life.

I want to focus on You.

Thank You for keeping me in a place of peace.

I love You.

Amen.

The Parental Prayer

Dear Father God,
Thank You for the blessing of bringing this baby
into this home.
Thank You for the excitement and anticipation
that is overwhelming me.
Please help me prepare
for the arrival of this new little one.
Help me to trust in You during this time of waiting
and draw me close to Your heart.
Help me to be the parent that You want me to be.
Show me how to be Your love here on earth to this child.
Be my strength when I am weak and
forgive me when I am wrong.
Please bless my marriage and grow it strong in You.
Lord, fill this baby to the top with
Your love, mercy, peace, and forgiveness.
Give me wisdom and patience, grace and understanding
for this new baby in full measure.
I commit this precious baby and our family into Your care.
Thank You for this new season of parenting.
Amen.

Chapter 38

Taking Care

THE BIG DAY is rapidly approaching. Your bag is packed. Your heart is ready. Your body is definitely ready. You will soon find yourself taking care of one of the most precious people in the entire world. Your child. And it is an around-the-clock job. It will require all of you to be up to the task. But you should know that there is one other person you are going to need to take special care of in the coming days. That person is you.

Now is the time to think a little about how you can care for yourself after the baby is born. It is easy to get lost in the wilds of post-partum after your labor and delivery. Everything is new. Your hormones are going nuts. You are trying to feed someone . . . with your body. You are sleep deprived. You are healing and recovering. It is okay to realize that you may need a few days or a month or more (like a year) to get up to speed. Every mom is wired differently. What you need during this time of recovery may not be what your best friend or your mom or your sister needed. But that's okay. You are unique. How you take care of yourself will be unique, too.

I found out that I desperately needed sleep and some alone time for my recovery. I had about seventy-three people who wanted to come visit me in the hospital the day after I had my first baby. Around visitor number sixty-two, I had a nervous breakdown. I was exhausted. I wasn't just learning how to take care of my baby. I was learning how to take care of myself so I could be a good mom. When I had baby number two, I kept hospital visitors to a minimum. I even got in a couple of naps. It was a win all the way around. My sister-in-law, Cheri, was the complete opposite of me. Visitors energized her. So she invited as many people as she could to visit her in the hospital. It made her feel loved. Cheri's hospital room was party central. It was exactly what she needed to recover.

Nurturing a new baby can be all-encompassing. Figuring out how to nurture yourself at the same time can be hard. But your heavenly Father is just as concerned about your well-being as He is about the well-being of your beautiful baby. He cares for you wholly. Your body, your mind, and your spirit. You are so precious to Him. When you have this little one, He will be cheering you on, bringing strength and healing, covering you with His peace. He is the One who said, "Love your neighbor as yourself." Loving yourself, taking care of yourself, enables you to love those around you even better. And know that both you and your baby are, even now, wrapped in the nurturing care of your heavenly Father.

Lord,
Thank You for the coming joy of caring
for this little baby.
Help me to know how to care for myself, as well.
Thank You for Your blanketing peace.
Amen.

Sweet Dreams

As the stars start to peep and the sun melts away
As the twilight grows dark at the end of this day
Keep my sweet baby safe in Your care
Tucked in Your mercy and wrapped warm in prayer

As the moonbeams shine bright and the nighttime
    breeze blows
As the cricket sings songs and the lightning bug glows
Lift my sweet baby close to Your face
Filled with your peace and bathed in Your grace

As the silver stars shine and my sweet baby dreams
As the evening air cools and the midnight moon beams
Give my sweet baby dreams from above
Soaked in Your goodness and drenched in Your love

Amen.

Chapter 39

The Good Mom

BECOMING A MOM is one of the most amazing things that can ever happen to you. The feeling of that little one in your arms, the sweet smell of their tiny head, the sight of their perfect little fingers and toes? It's almost too much for you to take in. And then there is the other side of becoming a mom. The part where you realize you are responsible for this tiny person for the next eighteen years. Protecting them, nurturing them, meeting their every need. That, also, can be almost too much for you to take in. The most pressing question you are probably asking yourself is . . . will you actually be a good mom?

When I brought Jack home from the hospital, my mom came to stay with me for three weeks. She helped me bathe him, rock him, and take care of him. When she left I thought I might die. *Where is she going? Doesn't she know that I have no clue what I am doing?* I had never raised a person before. She had raised four people. She was the good mom. If she could just stay with us until college, I thought I could take it from there. My mom came to stay with me each time I had a baby. Each time she left, I bawled like a baby. I'm sure this made Scott feel terrific. But the best mom I knew was walking out the door.

How in sweet heaven's name was I going to manage without my mom? Somehow it happened. *Managed* is the operative word here. There were some crazy days with my babies. Days of tears and no showers. Days when I thought, *Nope, I just cannot get out of bed* . . . I was so tired. But there were also high days of joy. The days of first smiles and giggles. The moments when only my arms would soothe their cries. And I started to figure out their cries. Each baby was so different. Different temperaments and personalities. Different wants and needs. But I learned them. I am learning them still. And the biggest lesson I learned? Those babies were made for me, and I was made for them. God had planned for me to be their mom. I was exactly the mom they needed.

As you are anticipating the arrival of this baby, you should know that there is no perfect mom. But your heavenly Father has found you to be the perfect fit for your little one. This doesn't mean that you will know everything or never make a mistake. It means that you are crafted to be the one who cares for this baby. You will learn what she needs and what she wants. And when you hold her close, soothing her cries, covering her with kisses, you will be doing exactly what God intended you to do. Loving her like no one else in the world could ever love her. You are the good mom.

Lord,

I believe that You created this baby for me
and me for this baby.

Guide me with Your wisdom and remind me
that I can lean on You and Your strength as
I learn how to be this baby's mom. I love You.

Amen.

Mommy's Prayer for Baby

Daddy's Prayer for Baby

Chapter 40

Hello, Love!

THE DAY YOU HAVE BEEN WAITING so long for is finally here. Baby Day! All of the days leading up to this day have been worth it. Even the nauseated, tired, and cranky days. The aching back and swollen feet days. The weepy, I-am-not-sure-I-can-do-this days. Because you are going to get to hold the most beautiful baby in the entire world today. This long pregnancy journey has come to a close, and all the light and joy of new motherhood is about to be yours.

Nothing could have prepared me for the moment of holding my baby for the first time. After twenty hours of labor, the midwife lifted Jack up and said, "It's a boy." And I burst into tears. Because I was a mom. His tiny cries filled the room as they gave him a quick wipe-down and cleared his lungs. And then the nurse placed him on my chest. I wrapped him in my arms and felt the warmth of his tiny body against mine. Scott leaned down to put his face near ours, and we all cried together. Me, Scott, and Jack. This new family. It was meant to be. We were bursting at the seams with love for each other. Scott picked Jack up and nuzzled his face. This was our son. Our beautiful son. We experienced those same breathtaking emotions when both Will and Addison were born. That high joy. The unprecedented, heart-wrenching love. The sense that we were living out a miracle. That we were seeing the hand of God hovering over this new baby. So lovely and fresh from heaven.

There really aren't words to describe the beauty of the moment when your baby is laid upon your chest. Nothing compares to what you feel when the warmth of this new life is filling your arms and your heart to bursting. There is the utter delight of joy of hearing your baby cry, filling its lungs with air, and hearing the doctor say, "It's a boy!" or "It's a girl!" The tears of joy and the threads of hope that lace themselves through your heart can't begin to express all that you are feeling. This is a great day. Your best day.

But I don't think it can compare with the party that is going on in heaven. This baby so lovingly crafted and knit together inside your body is making its entrance into the world. The angels are shouting with joy. There is dancing and singing. And your heavenly Father is celebrating. Big-time. He has to be. This little one whom He created with great love and with purpose and grace is fulfilling his destiny. His journey. Her journey. It is just beginning. And His good, sweet love for this baby is filling the room as you hold your little one close. It is a holy moment. Your baby is precious. The apple of his heavenly Father's eye. And He has entrusted this baby to your care. Bask in the joy of it. Soak it up. And know that as your mom adventure begins, He will be with you every single step of the way. Holding you close to His heart and wrapping you in His arms. Just like you are holding your baby. Hello, love.

Lord,
Thank You, thank You, thank You for this baby.
I am beyond thrilled to be this baby's mom.
You have given me the greatest gift.
Keep us close to You and wrapped in Your love.
Amen.

Hello, Love!

Baby's Name: _____

Date of Birth: _____

Time of Birth: _____

Baby's Height: _____ Baby's Weight: _____

Place of Birth: _____

(photo of your new sweet baby)

ABOUT THE AUTHOR

Susanna Foth Aughtmon is the mother of fourteen-year-old Jack, twelve-year-old Will, and nine-year-old Addison and the wife of Scott, the lead pastor of Pathway Church, in Redwood City, California. Their family has been church planting for nine years. Susanna has led worship, worked in children's ministry, and done the odd janitorial job here and there during their ministry.

In 1994, she graduated from Bethany University, in Santa Cruz, California, with a BA in social science emphasizing psychology and early childhood education, pursuing a career working with children before leaving to become a full-time mom and writer. She loves connecting with fellow Christ followers through her books and speaking using humor and the focus of how God's grace intersects our daily lives.

Susanna has written *All I Need Is Jesus and a Good Pair of Jeans: The Tired Supergirl's Search for Grace*, *My Bangs Look Good and Other Lies I Tell Myself: The Tired Supergirl's Search for Truth* and *I Blame Eve: Freedom from Perfectionism, Control Issues and the Tendency to Listen to Talking Snakes*. She co-wrote *Chasing God* with Roger Huang, *Need You Now* with singing artist Plumb, *A Trip Around the Sun* with Mark Batterson and Richard Foth, and *One Dress. One Year.* with Bethany Winz. She has contributed to Guideposts *Mornings with Jesus Devotional* 2013–16 editions. She blogs regularly at http://tiredsupergirl.blogspot.com.

IF YOU ENJOYED THIS BOOK, WILL YOU CONSIDER SHARING THE MESSAGE WITH OTHERS?

Mention the book in a blog post or through Facebook, Twitter, Pinterest, or upload a picture through Instagram.

Recommend this book to those in your small group, book club, workplace, and classes.

Head over to facebook.com/SusannaFothAughtmon, "LIKE" the page, and post a comment as to what you enjoyed the most.

Tweet "I recommend reading #ExpectantBlessings by Susanna Foth Aughtmon // @worthypub"

Pick up a copy for someone you know who would be challenged and encouraged by this message.

Write a book review online.

Visit us at worthypublishing.com

twitter.com/worthypub

facebook.com/worthypublishing

instagram.com/worthypub

worthypub.tumblr.com

pinterest.com/worthypub

youtube.com/worthypublishing